WALK YOURSELF WELL

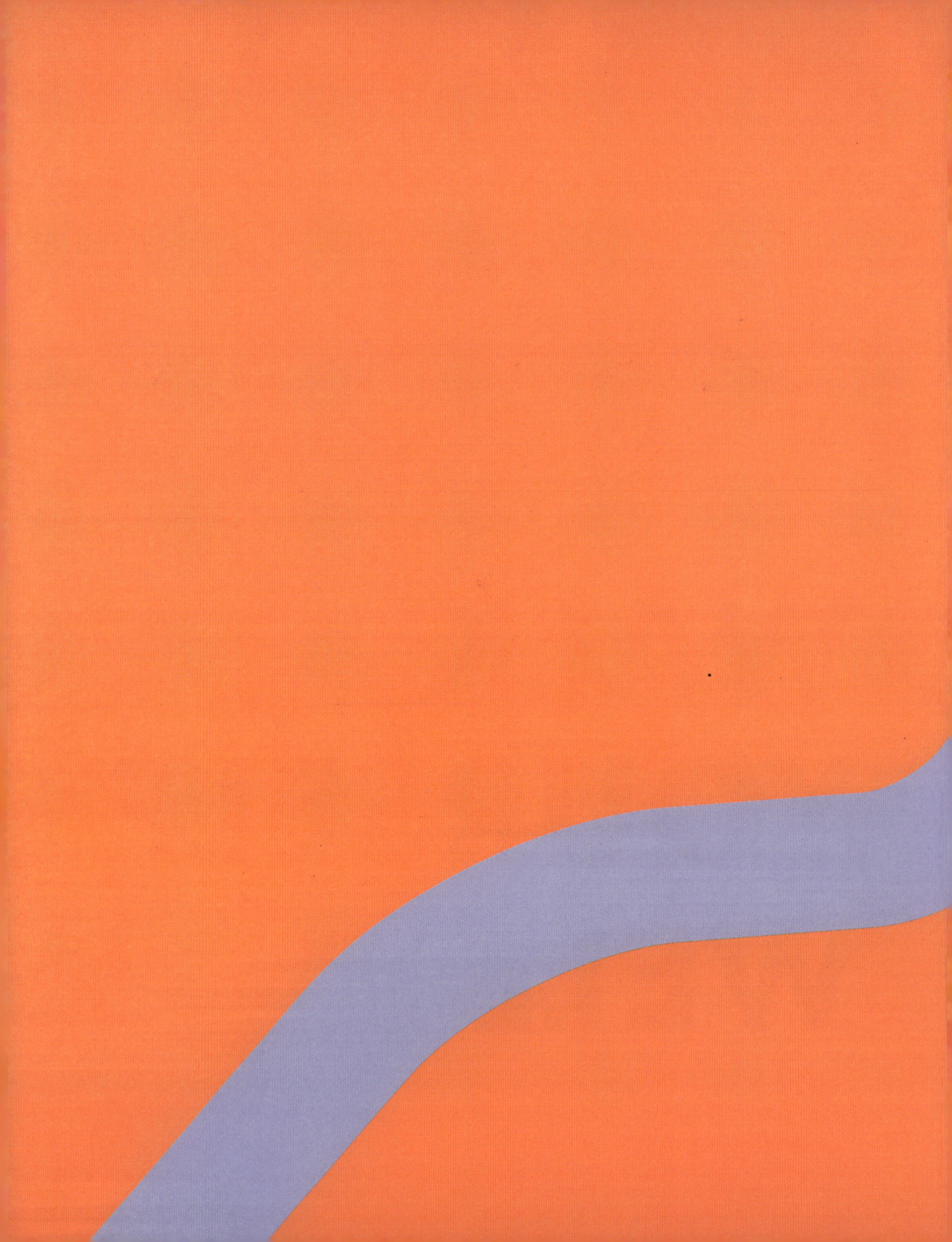

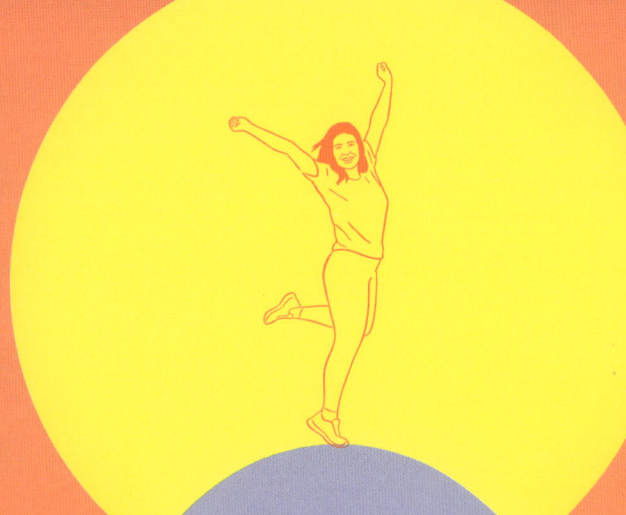

WALK YOURSELF WELL

Step into a healthier, happier you

NINA BAROUGH

Contents

Introduction 7

1. Why we walk 14

Walking for weight control 16
Walking for fitness 18
Walking for longevity 20
Walking for mental health 24
Walking at any age 26
Walking for pregnancy 28
Walking for children 30
Walking to heal 32

2. Getting started 34

The right shoes for you 36
Injuries 44
What to wear 46
Walking in different climates 50
Walking technology and accessories 52
Safety 54
Planning your route 56

3. Mastering your technique 58

Posture 60
Legs 62
It's all in the arms! 64
Putting it all together 66
Common mistakes 68
Staying injury-free 70

4. Stretch and strengthen 74

Why stretch and strengthen? 76
Stretches for beginners 78
Developing core strength 80
Upper body stretches 84
Lower body stretches 86
Full body stretches 88
Before and after walking 90
Warm up and cool down routine 94
Stretch and strengthen routine 95

5. Caring for your mind and body 96

The power of breath 98
A positive mindset 102
Be body aware 104
How to massage your feet 106
Foot care 108
The importance of water 110
Healthy choices 112
Vitamins and minerals 114
Foods for health and fitness 116

6. Ways to walk 120

Road walking 122
Treadmill walking 124
Hiking 126
Mindful walking 128
Rucking 130
Barefoot walking 132
Nordic walking 134
Competitive race walking 136
Challenge walking 138
Healthy walking 140

7. Training programmes 142

A daily walk 144
Walking yourself well 148
Weight control and fitness 152
Intermediate: muscle strength
    and stamina 156
Full marathon 162
Advanced: long distances, hikes,
    and challenges 168
Ultra fitness 174
Cross training 180

Walking log 182
Resources 184
References 185
Index 187
Acknowledgements 190
About the author 192

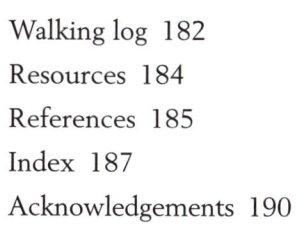
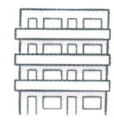
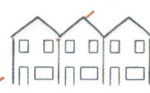
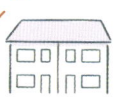

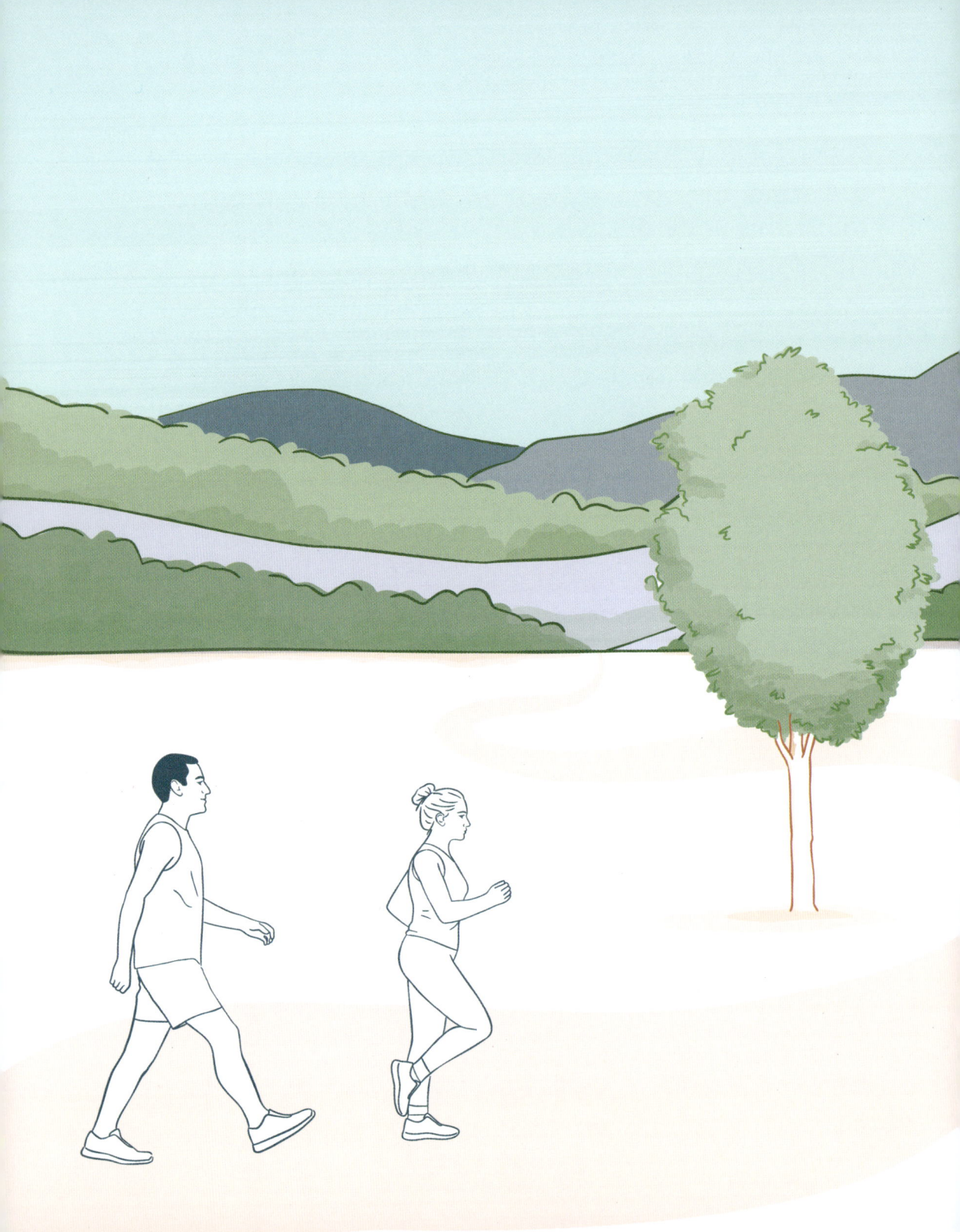

Introduction

There is strong evidence that whatever your age, staying physically active and walking are no longer something we should see as a choice. They are an essential part of being human, and leading a healthy and happy life.

From my own experience, walking has always been there for me, through wonderful times of trekking around the world, completing marathons, and Sunday walks with my family. It's also been there at some of my most challenging times, not least of all my journey through breast cancer.

During this stressful time, taking my daily walk inspired Walk the Walk, the cancer charity that I founded several decades ago. At that time, scientists knew that being active was important. However, they had no idea to what extent. Today, as our lives become more and more sedentary, there has never been more urgency to get up and get walking.

In this book you will discover the astounding number of benefits that come with something you do every day and so many of us take for granted. You will learn not only how your body works, but also how simple changes can have a huge impact on your health, fitness, and quality of life – all by putting one foot in front of the other.

If you are reading this, then you are one step closer to discovering the transformative benefits of walking and making it a part of your daily life. I really hope this book will open your eyes to what walking could do for you.

There are so many different ways to walk, from mindful walking and Nordic walking to rucking and training for a marathon, which you'll learn more about in this book. It can be energizing or relaxing, sociable or me time, exciting or calming, adventurous or wonderfully familiar, mindful or fun, but above all rewarding and nurturing. Regardless of your age, health, or fitness ability, everyone can benefit from walking, you just need to find a way that works for you.

I love walking. I love how it makes me feel. I love the many different ways I can walk, and I hope after reading this book, that you will love it too!

Love walking, love life!

> "Today, as our lives become more and more sedentary, there has never been more urgency to get up and get walking."

How fit are you?

Assessing your overall fitness, and regularly testing your abilities, including muscle strength, flexibility, and balance, is a good habit to have at any time. It helps you to keep a check on your health and gauge a starting point. As you progress, you can reasses your goals.

Your physical health depends on key factors such as aerobic capacity, muscle endurance, strength, and flexibility. Body composition, including bone and muscle mass and a healthy level of body fat, also plays a role, as well as diet and hydration. Monitoring these factors can help you set realistic, achievable goals that are suitable for your fitness capacity. Walking is an activity you can do every day to boost these areas. So whatever your goal, try completing 5,000 "AM–PM" steps: counting each step from the moment you wake up until bedtime.

FLEXIBILITY AND STRENGTH TESTING

There are simple ways that you can test your overall fitness at home, while taking into account key factors such as your age, gender, and level of fitness. Simple tests can include:

Flexibility Reaching to test your lower back and hamstrings (see box).

Balance and agility Standing on one leg for 30 seconds and then changing; rising up onto your toes, holding the position for the count of 10, closing your eyes for the count of 10 and repeating.

Upper body and core strength How many push ups can you do in 1 minute? Start from the classic push up position, or from your knees as an easier option.

Walk a mile Plot a 1 mile (1.6km) route. Using a stopwatch, walk at a pace that slightly increases your heart rate, but still allows you to talk. Good: 15–17 minutes; Average: 18–20 minutes.

Lower back flexibility test

To maintain a healthy back, test the flexibility in your lower back and hamstring muscles. Sit on the floor with your legs straight in front of you, ankles flexed, and feet flat against a wall. Reach your hands towards the wall. If your palms reach flat against the wall, your flexibility is excellent. Being able to place your knuckles to the wall is good; fingertips is average; not being able to reach at all means you have some work to do!

HEART RATE AND EXERTION

When you start any activity, it's important to know your aerobic fitness capacity, so that you work within safe and controlled levels of exertion. Your resting heart rate is a good guide to your current level of fitness. The stronger your heart is, the more blood it can pump through the body with each beat, which means it needs to beat less at rest, and while exercising, compared to the heart of an unfit person. To measure your resting heart rate, use your smart watch or a heart-rate monitor. A strap-on heart-rate monitor is the most efficient way of checking your heart rate while you are on the move.

Most adults have a resting heart rate of 60–100 beats per minute (bpm). The heart of an average fit adult beats at about 72 bpm at rest, and an unfit person often has a resting heart rate of 80–90 bpm. Some people naturally have a higher or lower heart rate.

Once you know your resting heart rate, you can establish what your optimum training zone should be. If you are unfit, you should work at the lower end of your maximum heart rate (MHR); if very unfit, you may need to drop as low as 55–50 per cent of your MHR. To work on your fitness, increase the intensity within the range of your training zone.

HEART RATE TRAINING ZONE

To work your heart and lungs in the most efficient way, it is important to exercise between 65 per cent and 85 per cent of your maximum heart rate (MHR).

If you are a man, 220 - your age = MHR

If you are a woman, 226 - your age = MHR

For example, if you are a 40-year-old woman, your MHR is 186 beats per minute (bpm).

To find your optimum training zone, work out the upper and lower limit percentages:

- 65 per cent of 186 (0.65 x 186) is 120 bpm

- 85 per cent of 186 (0.85 x 186) is 158 bpm

The training zone for a 40-year-old woman, therefore, is between 120 bpm and 158 bpm.

Working out above the upper limit would put unnecessary and unproductive stress on your body. Below the lower limit, you may not be working hard enough and may not see any real benefit from your walking programme.

Meeting your goals

Having established your starting point of fitness, how do you now achieve success? Begin to collect your toolkit of information on how to reach your goal. Break it down into small manageable steps that can fit into your life. Consider what technique or equipment may help you, and also any obstacles that you might encounter.

THE BORG SCALE

The Borg scale (see below) relies on your own perception of how fatigued or not you feel while exercising, particularly your muscles and level of breathlessness. It is therefore a quick way of assessing how hard you are working. It is useful for those that are at a high level of fitness and very aware of their bodies. Beginners may overestimate and assess that they are working harder than they really are. A person of average fitness walking at a brisk pace would likely feel they are working between 4 and 7 on the Borg scale. While it is subject to individual interpretation, the key is to be guided by how you feel. If you are working too hard, then slow down; if the workout feels too light, try stepping it up.

SETTING YOUR STRIDE

Your normal stride is largely set by the length of your legs. However, flexibility in your lower back, mobility in your hips, and flexibility in your hamstrings – the muscles at the back of your thighs – all play a part.

When it comes to walking, you may need to change your usual stride to meet the technique – optimal stride length can change depending on the type of walking that you are doing. Power walking requires keeping to your natural gait. Beginners often assume that if they take a longer stride they will move forward faster. In fact, the opposite is true. As you develop good technique, you naturally shorten your stride to take more steps per minute and by doing so move faster. By over striding, you become less

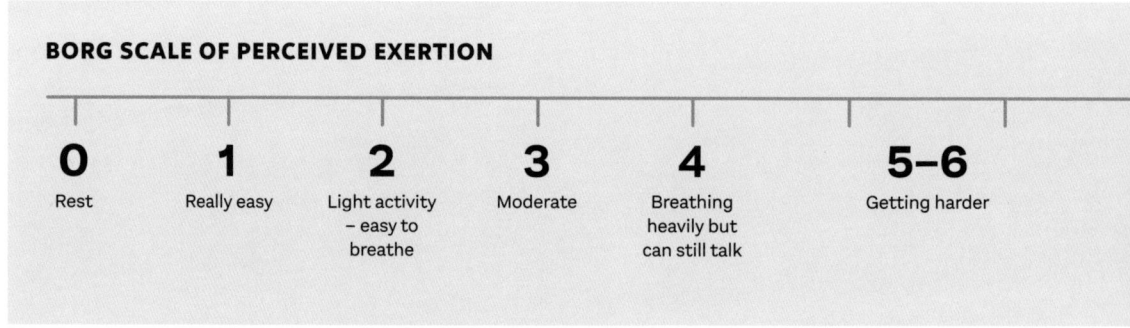

BORG SCALE OF PERCEIVED EXERTION

0	1	2	3	4	5–6
Rest	Really easy	Light activity – easy to breathe	Moderate	Breathing heavily but can still talk	Getting harder

stable, which indirectly slows your pace, and can cause injury. This is clearly demonstrated by race walkers. To reach the extraordinary speeds they do, their stride becomes shorter and very controlled. The transfer of weight from hip to hip is so quick they are only able to take small steps (see pp136–137).

Other types of walking, like Nordic walking, require a slightly longer stride for an effective workout and to minimize stress on the joints. However, because Nordic walkers use poles to propel themselves forward, the speed at which they walk is more a measure of their cardiovascular fitness than their stride length (see pp134–135). Proper technique, with continuous fluid movement, determines the ideal stride length for any type of walking you choose.

SETTING GOALS

It's exciting, it's life changing: you imagine that it's going to change everything. You suddenly decide you are going to get fitter, lose some weight for your holiday, or get that promotion at work. And then … life gets in the way, goals fall at the first fence and before you know it, it's history. Let's start again: the number one step to achieving any goal or ambition, is creating a good plan!

We all have dreams and dreams can come true. However, taking your dream from imagination to realization by setting a goal means you have made a decision that you are going to make it happen. For success, it must be achievable. Football coach Lou Holtz famously said, "It's not the load that breaks you down, it's the way that you carry it."

Step one, set your goal and make a solid plan. For example, if your goal is to walk a marathon, it will take a commitment of around 12 weeks, possibly more. You need time to build up to the necessary walking speed and stamina that will get you across the finish line. A walking plan will recommend how far, how fast, and when you need to walk each day (see pp162–168). Plot all the days into your diary as though they are meetings, which you are less likely to change or cancel. You might have to accommodate school runs, night shifts, or family holidays.

Step two, mark some major milestones into the plan. You may never have walked 5 miles before, or reached a certain speed. These will become your motivations and stepping stones to success. However many you have, be sure to celebrate each one, acknowledging what it means to you!

Step three is creating your safety net. If the going gets tough, you need a group of people you can turn to. There may be times when it all feels too hard, and you need to lean on someone who can remind you of your successes.

And finally, step four, don't try to go too fast, too soon. You have to be passionate about reaching any goal, and there will certainly be ups and downs that will try to throw you off course. These principles hold true for every area of your life and all your goals, so pace yourself both emotionally and physically, and success will be yours. Good luck!

7–8	9	10	*
Really hard, short of breath, talking in single sentences	Very difficult, hardly able to speak	Very very hard, unable to speak	Maximal

Fit walking into your day

Most of us live busy lives, so how can we possibly squeeze in something else? The beauty of walking is that you can do it anywhere and slot it in at any time. By simply being intentional about adding a few more steps to your day, you can boost your energy, mental clarity, and productivity, all without needing extra time.

How many times have you promised yourself, "Today's the day I'll start eating healthier" or "I'm finally going to get fit"? But life gets in the way, leaving no time to carry through those good intentions. Usually, work, children, or other commitments come first, leaving little or no time for ourselves. Yet if a friend asks for a favour, we can usually find the time to help. So, why are we never that kind to ourselves?

Instead of viewing walking as a task that you "have" to go and do, try seeing it as a purposeful activity as you move through your day, benefiting your health, mood, and fitness level. The rewards come fast, and quality is more important than quantity. A short, brisk walk to the corner shop can achieve more than a long, slow walk. For a busy person who feels finding the time to walk a few miles impossible, suddenly it becomes possible!

In truth, we can all find the time to do something if it is important enough to us. The secret is seeing the value that walking with purpose and being active every day can add to your life.

THE FIRST STEP

Start small. Knowing where to begin can feel daunting, especially if it's something you haven't done before, or you're doing it on your own. Focus on how you can naturally incorporate walking into your life, rather than making it something you have to add to an already busy schedule.

Wear a smart watch and start tracking an AM–PM plan so you can record the number of steps you take from the moment you get up in the morning, to going to bed at night. Get competitive with yourself and set daily targets, or try an online indoor workout. You can choose the time of day or night to suit you.

If you need a greater purpose to persuade you to take the first step, why not commit to a charity challenge? There is a multitude of both live and virtual events (see pp138–139). It's a great exchange, and you're not only improving your own health, but also raising money to help a good cause. You may even gather people motivated to join you.

Commit to walking in the very early morning, especially in the spring and summer; it's a great start to any day. Roll out of bed and go. Avoid checking any messages or socials. Set a time when you will make yourself available, but until then, allow yourself the free mind space to be in the moment. Whatever works for you, just start putting one foot in front of the other and see where it takes you.

PLOT SOME ROUTES

Choose a selection of pre-planned routes of various distances around your home area and work location so you won't have to think too hard about where to go, especially if you only have 15–20 minutes free (see pp56–57). Try to find routes that will include walking through parks or green spaces, and where there is little to no traffic. This will make them ideal for short bursts of interval training, or provide the space for mindful walks within a calming atmosphere, if you're in the midst of a busy day. Keep a spare pair of walking shoes and kit at work, so there really are no excuses for missing a chance to walk.

BOOK WALKING MEETINGS

By arranging "meetings" with yourself and adding them to your diary, you are more likely to work other commitments around them. As these "meetings" quickly become special "me time", you will be very reluctant to give them up. Why not arrange walk and talk meetings in your workplace? It is healthier for everyone; it has been proven to boost creativity and improve communications with those you work with. It also creates more walking time for yourself.

RECRUIT ALLIES

Having a walking buddy or like-minded person with a similar lifestyle to yourself can really make a difference. If you both have children, you can share childcare. If you work shifts, maybe you can meet others who want to walk at odd times such as late at night (see p55). Most areas have a local walking group, so when you don't feel like it, there will always be someone encouraging you to turn up. You could even form a group within your own network of friends. Make it a social event, work together on a training plan, and book a regular time and place to meet. Without a doubt, being part of a group is one of the best ways to make sure you stay motivated and keep walking (see pp26–27 and pp134–135).

FINDING TIME TO WALK

☑ Quality above quantity: enjoying a short walk is better than getting stressed by putting yourself under time pressures.

☑ Walk with purpose throughout the day: this even includes those shorts walks to the coffee machine.

☑ Be creative: walk all or part of the way when you would otherwise use transport.

☑ Be prepared: plot a few routes of different distances so you're always ready. Making it happen once is motivation for the next time.

☑ Arrange a meeting with yourself: put it in your diary, work around it, and learn how to say no to others.

☑ Join a walking group: form one of your own, or find a walking pal; shared activities are easier to manage.

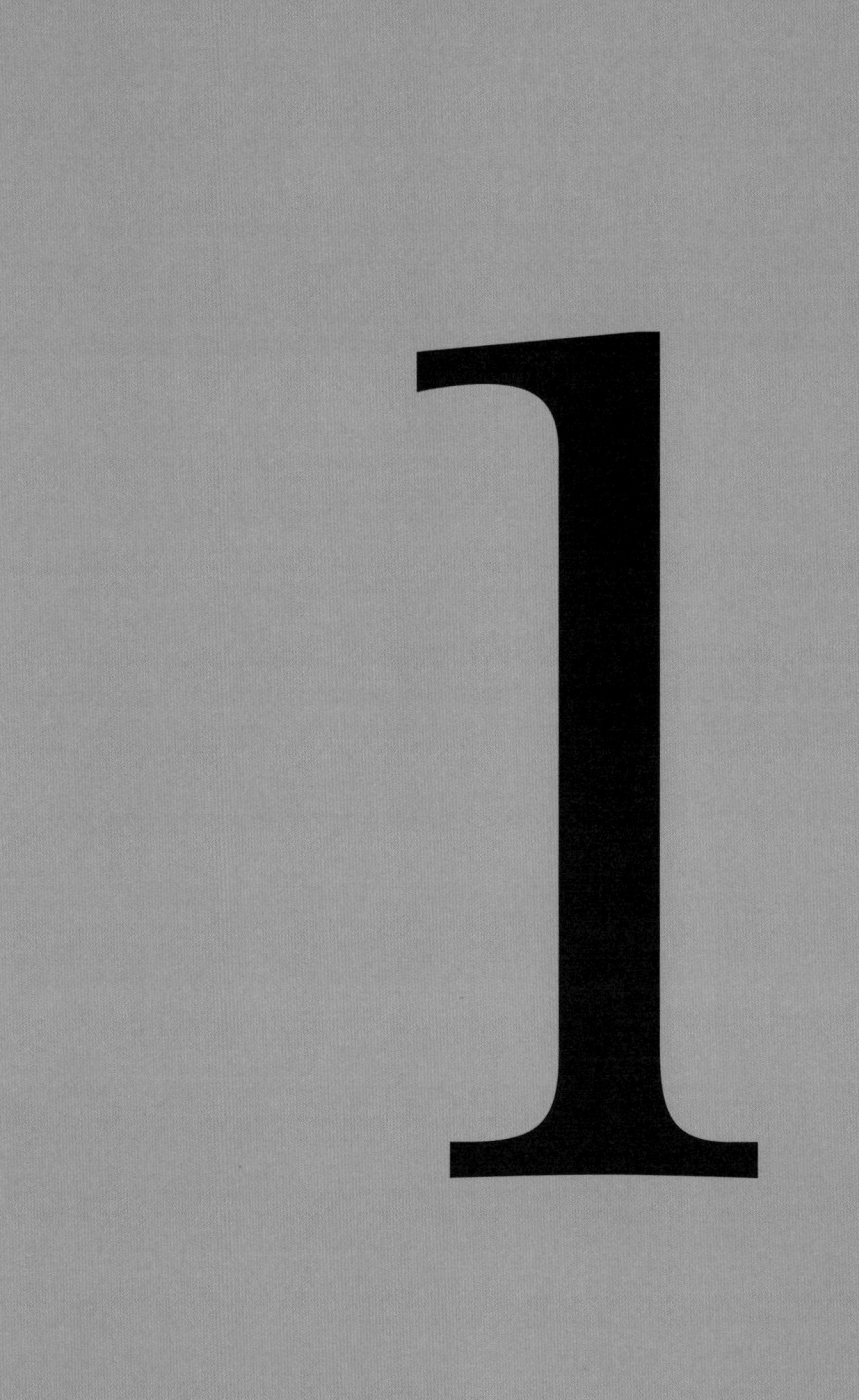

Why we walk

Why walk? It could be to get fitter and healthier, control your weight, develop muscle, find space to be mindful, or to care for your body during pregnancy. It could be a simple way to connect the generations in your family. Whatever your motivation, walking is an easy way to bring fitness to you, and everyone in your life.

Walking for weight control

When it comes to successful weight control, several factors come into play – no two people are the same – but commonly, it comes down to your diet, combined with activity levels, stress management, and sufficient sleep. Add stretching, strengthening workouts, and a few lifestyle changes, and you have all the tools you need to help you be a healthy weight.

It's not necessary to overdo it on the treadmill or in a spin class to lose weight healthily. Although walking is low impact, an average person walking four times a week for 45 minutes with an increased heart rate could lose around 8kg (18lb) within a year, without even changing their diet. Before starting, think about what you want to achieve and set some realistic goals.

Select a walking programme that aligns with your goals (see pp142–181) and start making adjustments to fit walking into your life. Treat your walks as special "me" time, or make them social. It's important that you see them as time to enjoy, not a hardship. Never weigh yourself more than once a week – or better still, go by how well your clothes fit.

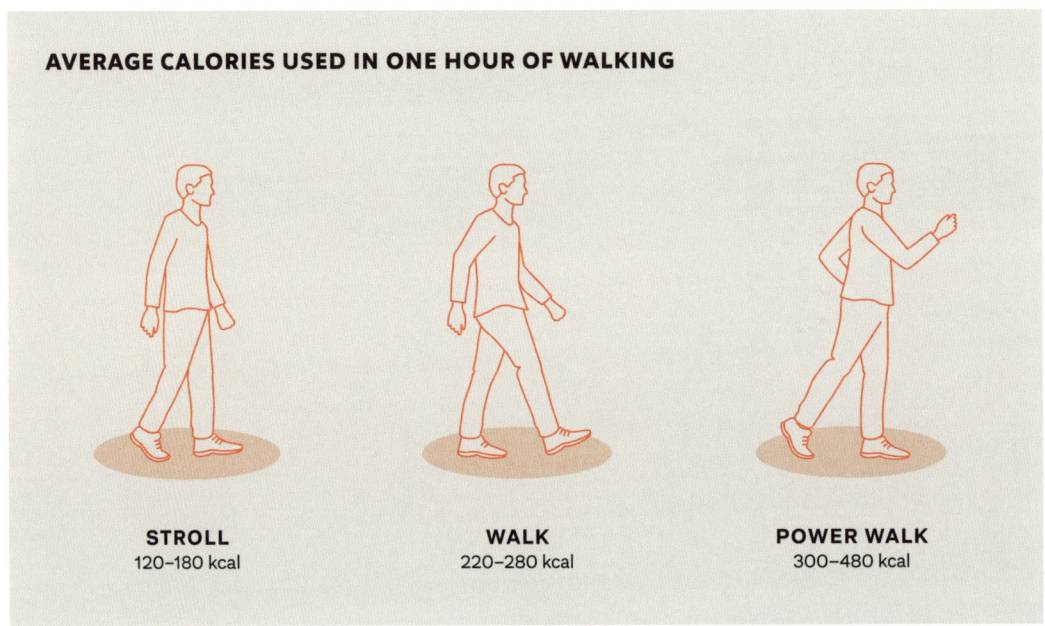

AVERAGE CALORIES USED IN ONE HOUR OF WALKING

STROLL
120–180 kcal

WALK
220–280 kcal

POWER WALK
300–480 kcal

AMP UP YOUR PACE

Aim to lose a maximum of 0.5–1kg (1–2lb) a week – any more and you will be losing water and muscle. Walking at a brisk pace burns approximately 300 calories an hour for the average person weighing 70kg (150lb). Increasing your heart rate by walking faster will burn more calories, especially if you are heavier. You may even find that there is no need to change your diet radically to lose weight, just reduce your intake and portion size.

BOOST YOUR METABOLISM

Introducing "intervals" – short bursts of fast walking in between periods of slower walking – is a great way to raise your aerobic level and speed up your metabolism. Walking builds muscle and the more muscle mass you have in ratio to fat, the faster your metabolism works. Your metabolic rate is the speed at which your body naturally burns calories or energy, even when sleeping. So not only will you lose body fat, you will also develop the muscle that will keep it off. Don't be disheartened if results are slow to begin with – this is normal, especially when you are combining lifestyle changes with exercise. Remember, you are building muscle, and muscle tissue weighs more than fat – so keep off the scales to start with!

> "An average person walking four times a week for 45 minutes could lose approximately 8kg (18lb) within a year."

INCREASE DISTANCE AND USE WEARABLES

It's worth noting that longer distances of at least 6km (4 miles) of active, uninterrupted walking (10,000 steps a day, depending on stride length and weight) are more effective for burning calories as well as improving strength. Using wearables and apps that are specifically designed to support weight control can map your routes, track your distance and step count, and monitor calories used. They will also track how much you actually do move throughout the day. It all adds up! Set a goal of 10,000 steps a day on your wearable – you'll be surprised at how it incentivizes you to meet that goal each day. As you gradually raise your pace and distance, use a heart-rate monitor to measure your optimum working levels.

WATCH THE CALORIES

Being aware of your calorie intake will help you plan your walking for weight control programme. Start by keeping a log and track absolutely everything you eat for a week. This can be revealing, especially if you're a snacker! Be honest with yourself at this stage, even if you may not like what your food log looks like. There are also apps that will keep your food diary, and offer advice and tips for when you feel like giving up. Many people now have access to what comprises a healthy and balanced diet, but beware: as you use more energy your appetite will grow. It's all a balance of calories in, energy out, so keep a check on what you eat (see pp112–119). Don't forget to drink plenty of water as dehydration can feel like hunger (see pp110–111), and always have plenty of delicious healthy food to hand for when you feel like raiding the fridge!

Walking for fitness

Can you get fitter "just" by walking? The answer in short is yes. If you're looking for a daily activity you can do anywhere that promises a toned body, lean muscle, a strong core, good aerobic fitness, balance and agility, flexibility, and a low risk of injury, along with a long list of other benefits, then walking is for you!

Walking engages all major muscle groups, especially those in your legs and core, and over time, it helps you build lean muscle and strength. Regular walking will help you maintain muscle mass as you age, regardless of your fitness level. If you follow a more intense training programme or add weights through rucking (see pp. 130–131), muscle development is likely to occur more quickly.

INTERVAL WALKING

You can do this by alternating between walking at a steady pace, followed by an intense burst of fast walking. The aim is to increase your speed for a set time (depending on your fitness) and then mirror this with a recovery pace. Initially you may need to walk at a recovery pace for longer. Use a smart watch to time yourself and repeat this cycle 4 or 5 times in a session, increasing as you progress. Intervals should be restricted to 1 or 2 sessions a week. A beginner's plan might look like this:

1. Warm up, walking at a moderate pace: 5 minutes
2. Walking briskly/fast: 30 seconds–1 minute
3. Walking moderately: 1–2 minutes
4. Cool down, walking a recovery pace: 5 minutes

Repeat 2 and 3 approximately five times.

POWER WALKING

Power walking is moving at a pace of 6–8kph (4–5mph). It is relatively easy to transition from being an average walker to a power walker. If you want to increase your speed, practising the right technique, and proper use of your arms is key (see pp64–65).

THE FIRST STEP TO FITNESS

Walking doesn't hold the philosophy of "no pain, no gain". Remember, you are in control of how much you walk and when. You may be suprised by how quickly you can progress and feel the difference just by walking for a minimum of 90–150 minutes a week, for two weeks. Regardless of the type of walk you choose (see pp122–141), the technique will remain the same – it is the intensity and goal that change.

Step one: put your shoes on and go for a walk at your own pace, short or long; see how good it feels.

Step two: turn to the technique pages and get practising (pp60–73).

Step three: walk again – this time taller, with a little more purpose.

MUSCLES TARGETED BY WALKING

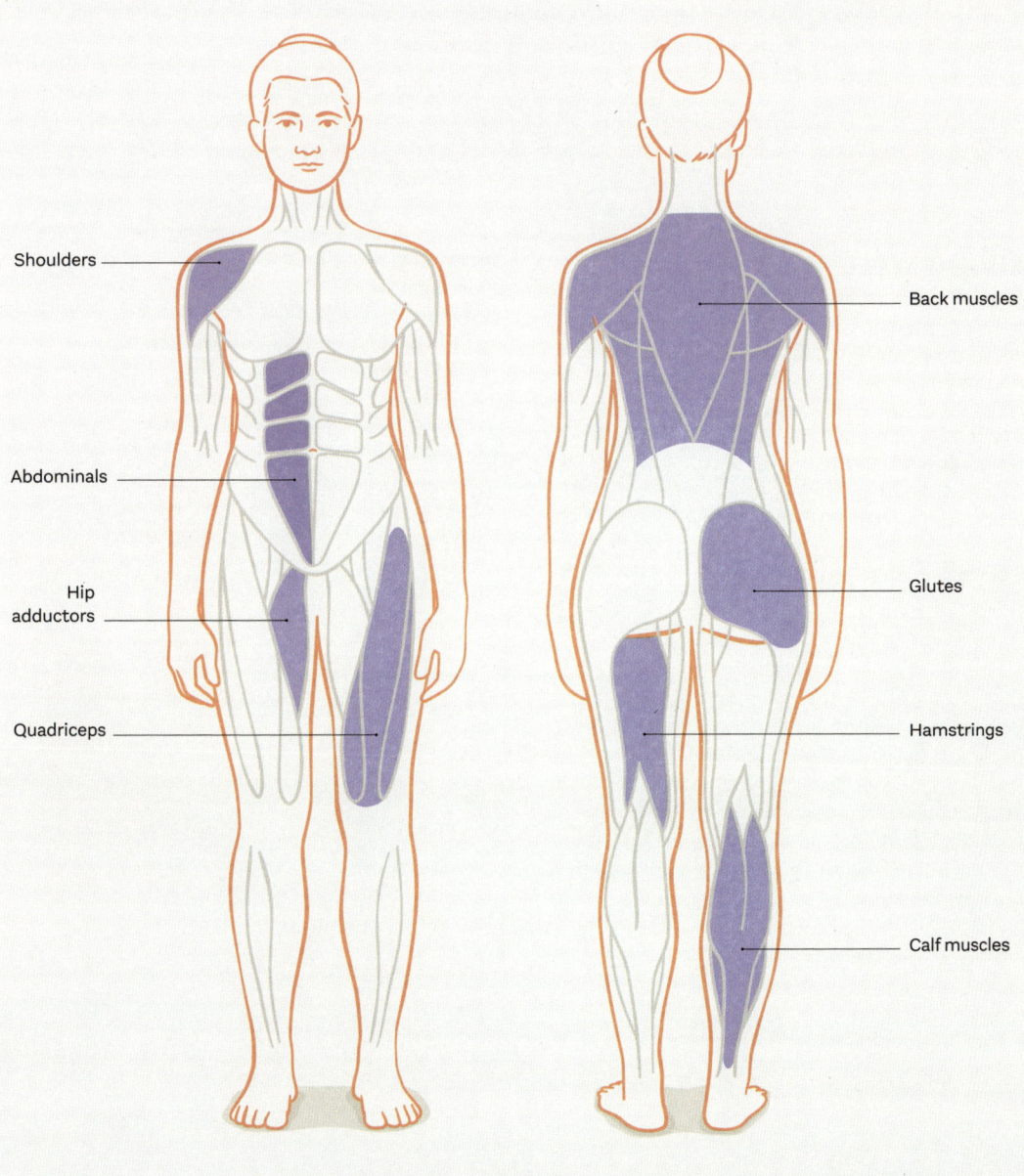

Walking for longevity

Today, the concept of longevity – living a long and healthy life – has become a hot topic. From promoting cardiovascular health to preventing disease, one fact is clear: walking regularly has a host of benefits that can support both the length and quality of life. Walking can also boost mental wellbeing and help maintain good cognitive function well into later years.

LIVING WELL

It's not just about living longer. Living well and having a good health span – the length of life a person spends in good health – are just as important. There are some interesting and revealing studies that are now showing how very simple lifestyle changes, such as staying active, might be the answer to a longer and healthier life.

MORE CENTENARIANS

It is interesting to see that centenarians – people who live to 100 years of age and beyond – are one of the fastest-growing age groups. With over half a million centenarians worldwide, this population is expected to grow eightfold by 2050. It is known that genetics only applies to 30 per cent of the difference in life span. So what about the other 70 per cent between centenarians, and the rest of us? As data is collected it is transforming the way that science thinks about health and ageing.

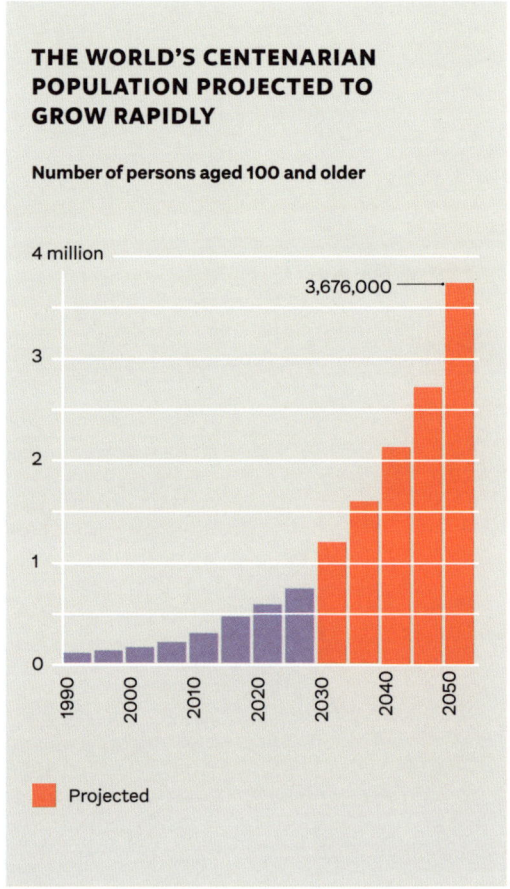

THE WORLD'S CENTENARIAN POPULATION PROJECTED TO GROW RAPIDLY

Number of persons aged 100 and older

THE POWER 9

Dan Buettner, a *National Geographic* Fellow and explorer, travelled the world looking for communities that not only had a record number of centenarians, but also of people living a long, happy, and high-quality life. He discovered five locations across the globe that he dubbed "Blue Zones": Okinawa, Japan; Ikaria, Greece; Nicoya, Costa Rica; Sardinia, Italy; and Loma Linda, California. While people lived differently in each zone, there were nine key commonalities all centred around their lifestyle, which he named "The Power 9".

1. Natural movement: With high levels of walking and continual low impact movement, people in the Blue Zones walk everywhere as part of their day-to-day routine. We should all try to move naturally as much as we can during the day, rather than saving activity for the gym.

2. Purposeful living: Having a purpose in day-to-day life and staying optimistic about the future gives these communities a reason to get up every day. A sense of purpose can add an extra seven years to your life, so it is worth doing some soul searching to discover yours.

3. Low stress: Even those living in the Blue Zones have stresses to deal with, but they learn to approach them in healthy ways – be it through meditation, praying, or even napping. Managing stress is essential, as it leads to chronic inflammation associated with every major disease, including heart disease, blood pressure, and cancers (see pp22–23).

4. Healthy body weight: A Confucian mantra called *Hara Hachi bu* intoned before meals reminds Okinawans to stop eating when they are 80 per cent full. This 20 per cent can be the difference between gaining or losing weight. People in the Blue Zone eat their smallest meal in the early evening, and then leave 12 hours before eating again.

5. Mainly plant-based diet: Blue Zone dwellers consume a diet that is 95 per cent plant based. This often consists of beans, lentils, soy, nuts, whole grains, and vegetables (see p116).

6. Moderate alcohol consumption: A glass of wine enjoyed with food and friends as a social activity emphasizes the role of community. A study showed that moderate drinkers lived longer than abstainers – it's better to share a glass every so often with food than saving all your drinking for the weekend and maxing out on your units in one day!

7. Strong, nurturing relationships: Investing in family and community is key in the Blue Zones. People live among all age groups, keeping ageing parents and grandparents nearby, and most commit to a life partner, which can add three years to their life.

8. Faith-based services and belonging: Most people living in a Blue Zone belong to a faith-based community. Regardless of denomination, belonging to any kind of group, especially in later years, can add length to your life.

9. Social circle: The longest-lived people choose positive social circles that support healthy behaviours. Find your tribe of people who bring you joy and stimulation.

DANGERS OF A SEDENTARY LIFESTYLE

Researchers at Queen's University, Belfast found that spending large amounts of time sitting or lounging around during the day is linked to around 70,000 deaths per year in the UK alone. Sedentary behaviour presents risks for developing type 2 diabetes, colon cancer, cardiovascular disease, endometrial cancer, and lung cancer. We know that eating foods rich in antioxidants can help reduce inflammation and eliminate waste products from the bloodstream, but walking has also been shown to have similar effects. The good news is that walking for just 20 minutes a day has a host of benefits to support longevity:

- By increasing your heart rate, improving your circulation, and lowering your blood presssure, walking can improve cardiovascular health, reducing the risk of heart disease by up to 30 per cent.

- Walking gets the blood circulating, helping your white immune-boosting cells move freely around the body. So it makes sense to walk as much as possible to protect from illness, especially during the winter months when colds and flu are prevalent.

- It can decrease your risks of getting some cancers; for women, walking lowers hormone levels that increase the risk for developing breast or endometrial cancers.

- It can reduce arthritis-related pain, especially in the knees and hips. Contrary to making arthritic pain worse, walking actually can help by strengthening the muscles around the affected joints.

"Sedentary behaviour is linked to around 70,000 deaths per year in the UK alone."

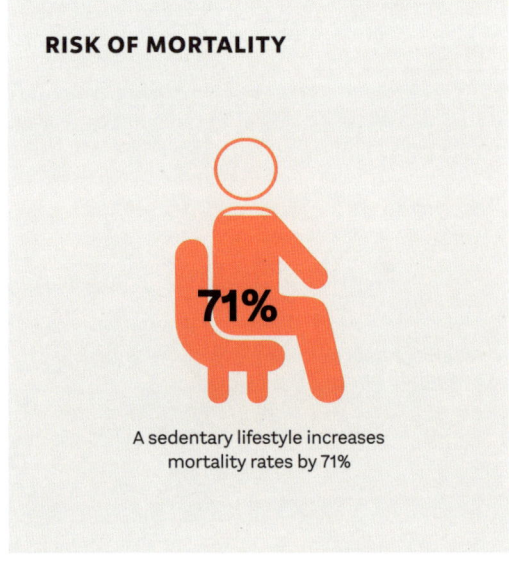

RISK OF MORTALITY

71%

A sedentary lifestyle increases mortality rates by 71%

KEEP ON MOVING

Walking is something many of us take for granted. It is the most accessible form of exercise and offers countless benefits that can improve both our health and overall quality of life. There is now scientific evidence suggesting that walking and staying active have healing and rehabilitation properties following illness. It also appears to be the panacea for prevention against disease (see pp32–33). Taking part in any kind of physical activity releases chemicals in the body known as neurotransmitters. These help prevent age-related diseases, making it an important factor of longevity.

MAKING THE POWER 9 WORK FOR YOU

We may not all be budding centenarians, but we can all improve our health by adopting a few of their simple principles. Hopefully this inspires you to consider introducing new and healthy habits into your daily life. Bad habits can be hard to break, and new ones hard to adopt, depending on how big the changes are. Be prepared, and stay patient – it can take several weeks and even months to fully embrace them. For this reason, only attempt two or three of the Power 9 at any one time, to give yourself the best chance of success!

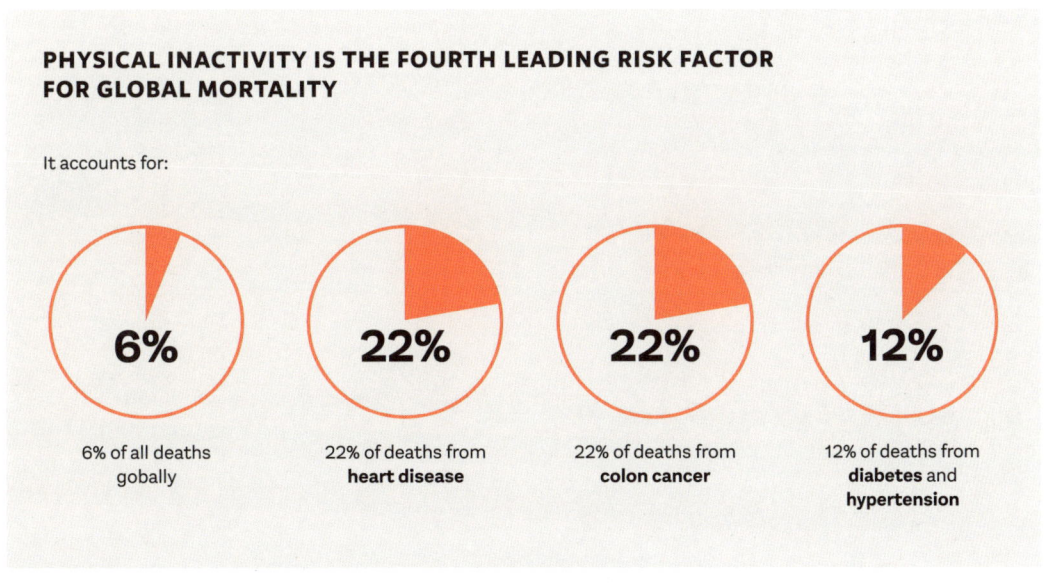

PHYSICAL INACTIVITY IS THE FOURTH LEADING RISK FACTOR FOR GLOBAL MORTALITY

It accounts for:

- **6%** — 6% of all deaths gobally
- **22%** — 22% of deaths from **heart disease**
- **22%** — 22% of deaths from **colon cancer**
- **12%** — 12% of deaths from **diabetes** and **hypertension**

Walking for mental health

Just a 10-minute walk in nature every day can have a powerful impact on our mental health and wellbeing. Those few minutes can lift your mood, reduce anxiety, increase your self-esteem and, by naturally releasing endorphins – "happy hormones" – promote happiness.

For years, medical professionals worldwide have acknowledged the link between physical activity and mental health. Doctors now commonly prescribe non-clinical interventions, or "green prescriptions", to help treat depression and anxiety. They recommend that staying active and spending time in nature, whether through walking, gardening, or part of community food-growing projects, can promote mental alertness, increased energy, and a more positive outlook.

WALKING WITH NATURE

The powerful impact that nature can have on our mental and physical wellbeing has been known for centuries. Walking in the great outdoors is an wonderful way to reap these benefits. The colour green, associated with nature, has been proven to have a calming effect, creating a sense of tranquillity. Celebrated architect Frank Lloyd Wright once said, "Study nature, love nature, stay close to nature. It will never fail you." While not everyone has easy access to green spaces, you don't need to go far – public parks, community allotments, and gardens can all offer the comforting and healing powers of nature. Researchers found that even owning a single plant could have a significant impact on stress and anxiety. Walking barefoot or standing on grass or soil – called "grounding" or "earthing" – can reconnect you to the earth and realign your electrical energy, by absorbing the earth's electrons. While the studies are small, the reports have shown it to have a calming effect on the body, as well as other healing benefits.

TIME IN NATURE

Reduces
- Depression
- Stress
- Anxiety
- Rumination

Increases
- Meditative feelings
- Good mood
- Empathy
- Attention and focus

A 90-minute walk in nature reduces negative self talk

BENEFITS OF WALKING FOR MENTAL HEALTH

Self-esteem and confidence: Walking has been proven to boost self-esteem, which in turn will reduce stress and improve social interactions and relationships.

Reduced risk of depression: In a study, 25 per cent of people who were walking briskly for the recommended time of 2.5 hours per week, had lowered risk of depression.

Improved sleep: Regular walking can make a big improvement on the quality and duration of your sleep. You will notice very quickly how your sleep pattern improves. We all need different amounts, but having enough sleep can make you feel more calm, in control, tolerant and patient, open to trying new things, and content.

Reduced stress: A sedentary or stressful job, or spending a lot of time inside, can cause an increase in cortisol (the "stress hormone"). Research shows that being active, walking regularly in fresh air, and being in nature can lower levels of cortisol and reduce stress.

Friendship and camaraderie: Walking with friends or in an organized group can combine being active with reducing loneliness through positive social contact. The combination of regular walking and the chance to have fun and build new friendships releases endorphins, making us feel good. The same hormones will also help you to have better concentration and feel mentally sharper in areas of your daily life.

> "You don't need to go far – public parks, community allotments, and gardens can all offer the comforting and healing powers of nature."

TIPS FOR STARTING WHEN YOUR MOOD IS LOW

- **Start small.** If you're in a fog of depression, set yourself doable goals and build up from there. Don't sign up for a charity walk just yet. Head out at a time of day when your energy is highest.

- **Reward yourself.** If you've completed a good walk, pat yourself on the back for getting out there. Have a relaxing bath or your favourite hot drink.

- **Be comfortable.** Wear clothing that feels comfortable and make sure you have the right-fitting shoes (see pp36–43).

- **Ask a friend.** Planning to walk with a friend or family members will make it more enjoyable and will also make you accountable on days you don't feel like leaving the house.

Walking at any age

As you head into your 70s and beyond, the thought of following an exercise programme like walking can be quite daunting – you may also wonder if it will do you any good! But the message from all the research bodies is clear: if you want to be as fit, healthy, and mobile as possible, well into older age, it is never too late to start.

Gaining confidence in your own physical ability allows you the freedom to make choices about how you live. You might want to join a walking group, which could give a real boost to your social life, or enjoy walking to a local café or pub. You could even consider having the companionship of a dog!

PROVEN BENEFITS

The list of benefits from regular walking is long, and the figures speak for themselves. Researchers found that older adults who walked faster than 5km (3 miles) per hour had a 50 per cent lower risk of heart disease than those who walked slower than 3km (2 miles) per hour. The practice also helps to retain muscle strength and, most importantly, mobility and balance, decreasing the likelihood of falling. It also helps with cognitive function – a study showed that adults who walked regularly had a 38 per cent lower risk of cognitive decline. Plus, it can ease anxiety and depression, which often leads to loneliness in later years.

HOW DO I START?

Given these statistics, the question should be not "if", but "how" to get started. Visit your doctor and ask them to assess any health issues, such as high blood pressure. Exercise is proven to reduce high blood pressure, but your practitioner may want to lower it with medication before you start.

It's estimated that adults of 69 and older, who are regularly active, could take 3,400 steps (113 steps per minute) during a 30 minute walk. Set yourself stepping-stone goals aiming for 2,000–9,000 every day. As an older walker, it can be beneficial to break up your daily goal into two or three shorter walks rather than one long one, but be sure to celebrate each stage you reach, and remember that something is always better than nothing.

"Walking helps to retain muscle strength, and, most importantly, mobility and balance."

WALKING GROUPS

Walking with a friend, or an established walking or "rambling" group has so many benefits for older adults.

- The commitment to the friend or group will get you out the door on days you may not feel like it.

- Chatting while walking makes the time fly by and you won't notice the distance you're covering.

- A walking group brings camaraderie, fun, encouragement, and support, as well as new friends, which together benefit both body and mind.

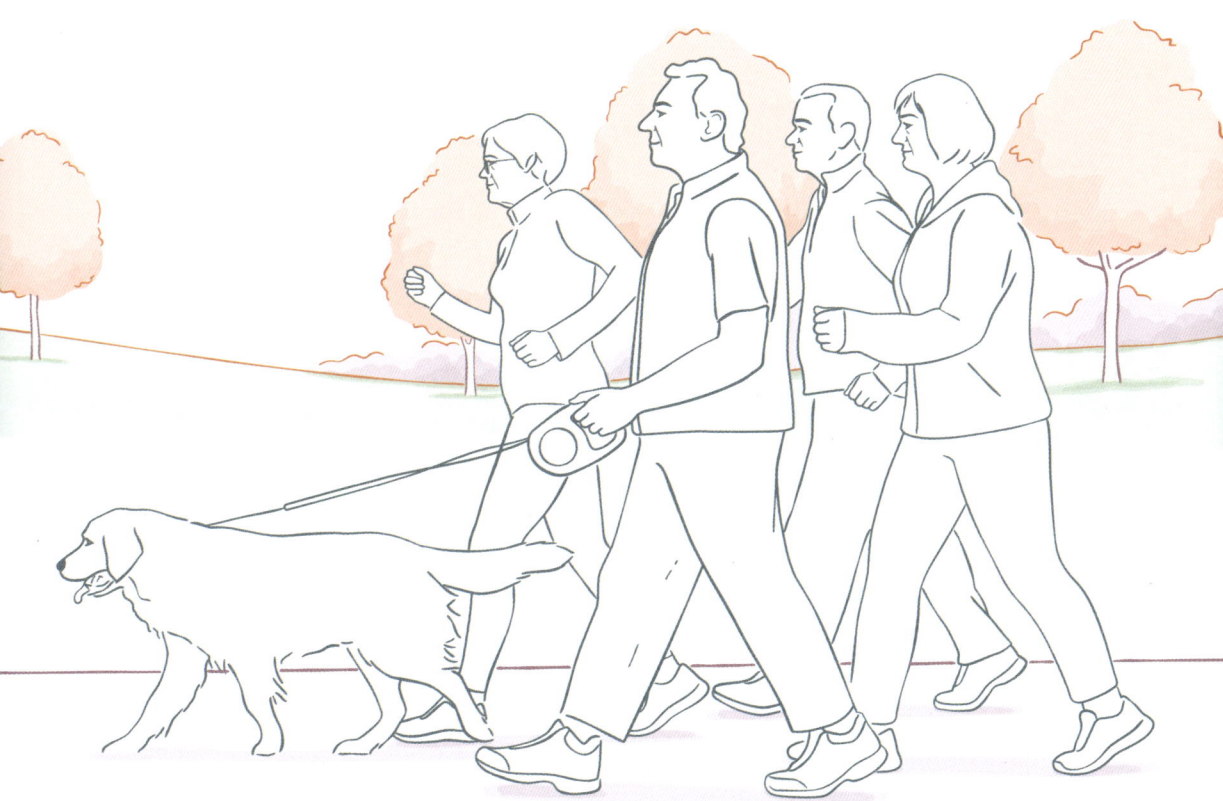

Walking for pregnancy

As a low-impact, cardiovascular exercise, walking will help to keep you fit, strong, and healthy from the first trimester through to the delivery of your baby. Before embarking on your walking journey, discuss any exercise plan with your doctor, particularly if you are new to the activity.

It has been proven that moderate activity during pregnancy can reduce the risk of complications such as pre-eclampsia, as well as irksome symptoms like back pain and constipation. Proceed with caution though – if you were fairly inactive or very unfit before becoming pregnant, you will need to build up your walking slowly. Aim to walk three times a week, building up to 20–30-minute sessions. Always keep yourself well hydrated (pp110–111), and plan your routes close to your home. If you do feel overtired or short of breath you can stop immediately.

WALKING METRICS IN PREGNANCY
Take shorter strides than usual, creating less aggressive movement in your hips. It is worth noting that during and just after pregnancy, your body releases the hormone relaxin, which

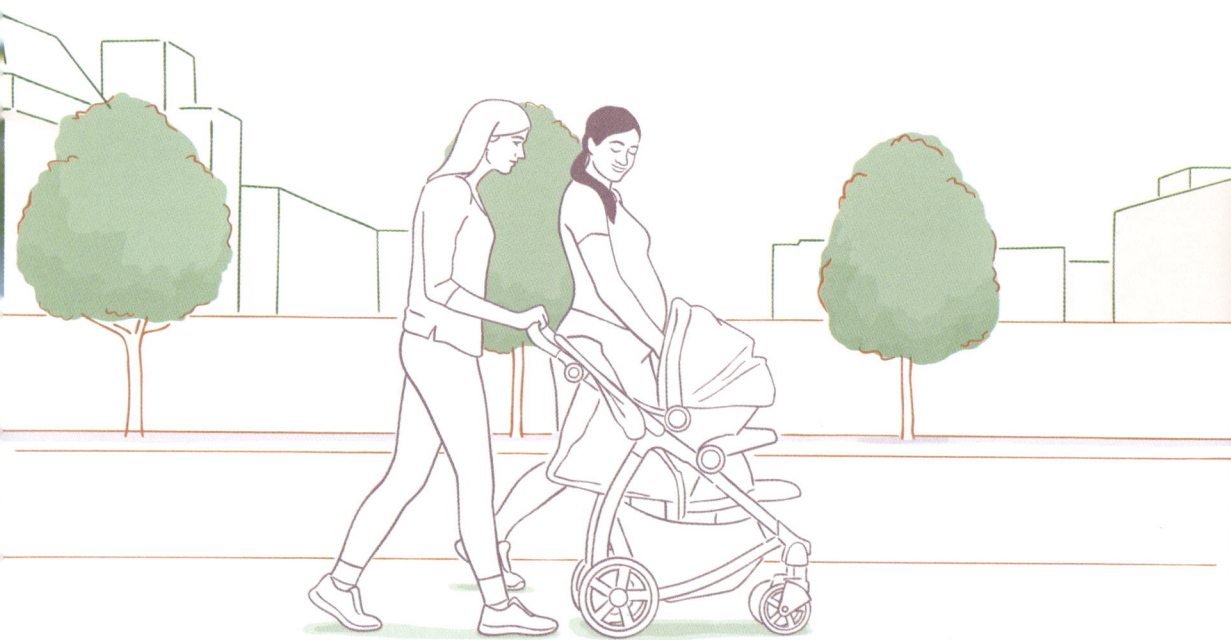

PROGRAMMES BY TRIMESTER

- *Trimester 1 (weeks 1–13):* You may feel exhausted or may be suffering from morning sickness, so take it slowly if this is the case. Even if you feel supercharged with energy, be mindful of the intensity of your walking. Also, keep cool and avoid walking in hot or humid weather, as overheating is not good for the baby.

- *Trimester 2 (weeks 14–26):* You might feel more energy and motivation to exercise in this trimester, but stay conscious of your posture to avoid straining your back (see pp60–61), remembering to look ahead. To avoid tripping, try to keep away from uneven ground such as trails and beaches – stay on the tarmac.

- *Trimester 3 (weeks 27–40):* Take note of how your centre of gravity has shifted with your expanding belly, and stick to flat paths to avoid tripping and falling. Never walk further than feels comfortable at this stage. Keep going for as long as you can, albeit at a slower pace and without pushing yourself. As your weight increases, your arches will be under more pressure and your feet may swell a bit. Check your shoes are supportive and comfortable; if necessary go up a half or full size.

softens and loosens your joints in preparation for childbirth. This newly found flexibility can lead to overextending, and while it may sound wonderful to be so agile, be cautious not to push your body.

AFTER THE BIRTH

After welcoming their baby to the world and going through the birth process, many women, as well as feeling overwhelmed, experience physical changes.

Diastasis rectus abdominis refers to the natural separation of the abdominal muscles vertically, which happens by the end of all pregnancies. Many women's abdomens return to normal after some weeks, but some experience a continuing weakness in the area. As well as gentle abdominal exercises (such as certain Pilates movements), regular walking is one of the best ways to heal this separation.

The pelvic floor comes under immense strain during pregnancy, and about 75 per cent of women experience pelvic floor dysfunction postpartum, including mild urinary incontinence. Walking strengthens and tones all the muscles that support your pelvic floor, and, in conjunction with pelvic floor exercises like tightening and releasing the area, will help train these muscles back into shape.

WALKING WITH YOUR BABY

Look forward to walking with your beautiful baby when they arrive – it's joyous! You could carry your baby with you in a carrier or use an all-terrain buggy, but keep an eye on your posture (see pp60–61). Keep your arms bent and push with your body weight, rather than just using your shoulders. If you have an older baby (6 months+) or toddler, carry them in a well-fitting backpack as it is better for your posture and overall technique.

Walking for children

Physical activity is vital for a child's healthy development, and the earlier it's introduced, the greater opportunity they have of developing strong motor skills. It can also support their academic achievements, mental health, and fitness. Walking can be introduced so easily into a child's life, whether it's getting to school, or walking for leisure.

For a child, every walk improves balance, posture, flexibility, and coordination, and boosts feelings of wellbeing. If parents are keen walkers from the start, their children will learn through example that walking should be an essential part of everyday life.

YOUNGER CHILDREN

Most younger children make excellent walking companions and will certainly walk further when there is something to see and do. Increase stimulation, learning opportunities, and fun by plotting routes through parks, streams, and woods, looking for wildlife, creating games, or taking paper to try some stencilling on your route. If you can add in a playground at some point, even better. Plus, the games and conversations that you share as you walk not only help to build and nurture their life skills; you are also sharing special times together.

HOW FAR?

As a guide to distance, estimate 1km (½ mile) per birthday, so a three year old should be able to walk 3km (2 miles), albeit at a slower pace, and with a few stops no doubt! For children over the age of five, 60 minutes of moderate to vigorous activity every day is recommended, including playing outdoor games and sports.

TWEENS AND TEENS

While a good game can get younger children out walking, convincing a teenager can be trickier. Most tweens' and teens' lives revolve around their friendship groups – they want to be independent and need a proper reason to do anything. The first step is prising them away from their tablets and phones, and probably not calling it "a walk".

With hormones raging at an extremely complex stage of their development, the rhythm of walking can be calming and reduce anxiety. Walking side by side can lead to open conversation, which can be challenging for teenagers. Being physically active releases feel-good endorphins that encourage mood stability, and any activity, regardless of what it is, that leads a teenager to focus on their health and fitness has to be considered a good thing.

It might be the last thing they want to do, but combining walking with visiting a destination such as the cinema, to meet a friend, or setting a distance to cover in a shopping mall will be a great start.

> "Walking side by side can lead to open conversation, which can be challenging for teenagers."

GROUND RULES

Always take plenty of water, favourite healthy snacks (such as flapjacks), and agree to all put phones in pockets, allowing the conversation and the steps to flow.

GEOCACHING TREASURE HUNTS

One way to get everyone walking and talking is Geocaching, a worldwide treasure hunt. The "caches" – cleverly hidden, small waterproof containers – usually hold a log book, pen or pencil, and some "treasure" – small items such as coins or badges. There are in fact, millions of "caches" across 190 countries in both rural and urban settings, so there is definitely one near you.

Like orienteering, all you need is a mobile phone, the free app, or use of a handheld GPS device to navigate the coordinates produced by the cache website. Locations can be as easy or as challenging as you want, and it's a great way for teens to take control and explore. When you find a "cache" you add your name to the log book and take a trinket, as long as you replace it with something of the same value. What could be more fun than searching for treasure?

TAKE A CHALLENGE

If you need to satisfy a competitive spirit, there are plenty of 5k and longer-distance charity challenges that are open to all ages and abilities (see pp138–139). The combination of building up to a challenge, raising money for a favourite charity, and coming away with a medal or T-shirt is sure to put a spring in any child or teenager's step.

Walking to heal

Hippocrates was right when he said, "Walking is man's best medicine." More than 2,000 years later, something we take for granted is now being prescribed by doctors as a treatment for both emotional and physical conditions. Strong evidence proves that regular exercise such as walking, before and as soon as possible after any surgery, leads to a faster recovery.

POST-SURGERY WALKING
It might seem counterintuitive for those recovering from surgery, but medical professionals like to get patients up from bed and walking around the ward as soon as possible after a procedure. Once you are encouraged to take that first step, it is the most accessible and effective form of rehabilitation, helping to reduce swelling, promote healing, and increase blood flow and mobility. It also leads to a faster recovery and fewer post-operative complications. In fact, Dr Thomas Frieden referred to walking (and other types of exercise) as the "closest thing we have to a wonder drug".

WALKING FOR CHRONIC DISEASES
For those who live with chronic diseases such as hypertension or diabetes, walking regularly will reduce blood pressure and blood sugar, as well as oxygenating the blood. For arthritis, walking can help sufferers gain flexibility and reduce joint stiffness. Similarly, osteoporosis patients can strengthen bones, reduce fracture risk, and improve bone density through walking.

WALKING DURING CANCER TREATMENT
Scientists have proven that the rigours of cancer treatment such as radiotherapy and chemotherapy can be eased by walking. The new understanding is that rather than curling up on the couch with a blanket post-treatment, a walk in the fresh air will bring many more benefits, helping with the symptoms like fatigue, anxiety, and depression that naturally accompany any kind of cancer journey. It will also give the patient a sense of empowerment, of taking control at a time when they feel that they have lost it.

"Dr Thomas Frieden referred to walking as 'the closest thing we have to a wonder drug'."

ACTIVE RECOVERY

These days, coaches will often tell athletes to "walk it off" after a small injury like a rolled ankle, rather than staying sedentary and icing the area. And after a tough workout, taking a 30-minute walk is the optimal way to bring breathing back to normal, increase blood flow, and relieve stiff muscles.

HOW MUCH SHOULD YOU WALK?

The answer to this question is unique to each person, and to the type of illness they are recovering from. It depends on your personal health, and factors that should always be first discussed with the doctor supervising your recovery. However, as a rule, always start small. To begin with, you may feel like you need the determination of an Olympic athlete to only walk around your home or climb the stairs. Be realistic with your expectations, because any walking is better than none. Whatever you were able to do today, no matter how small, try to do a little more tomorrow. It also helps if you have a friend who can join you. They can help with motivation on the tough days, inspiration as you begin to walk further, and the joy of laughter as you step out together ... healing and progress will follow!

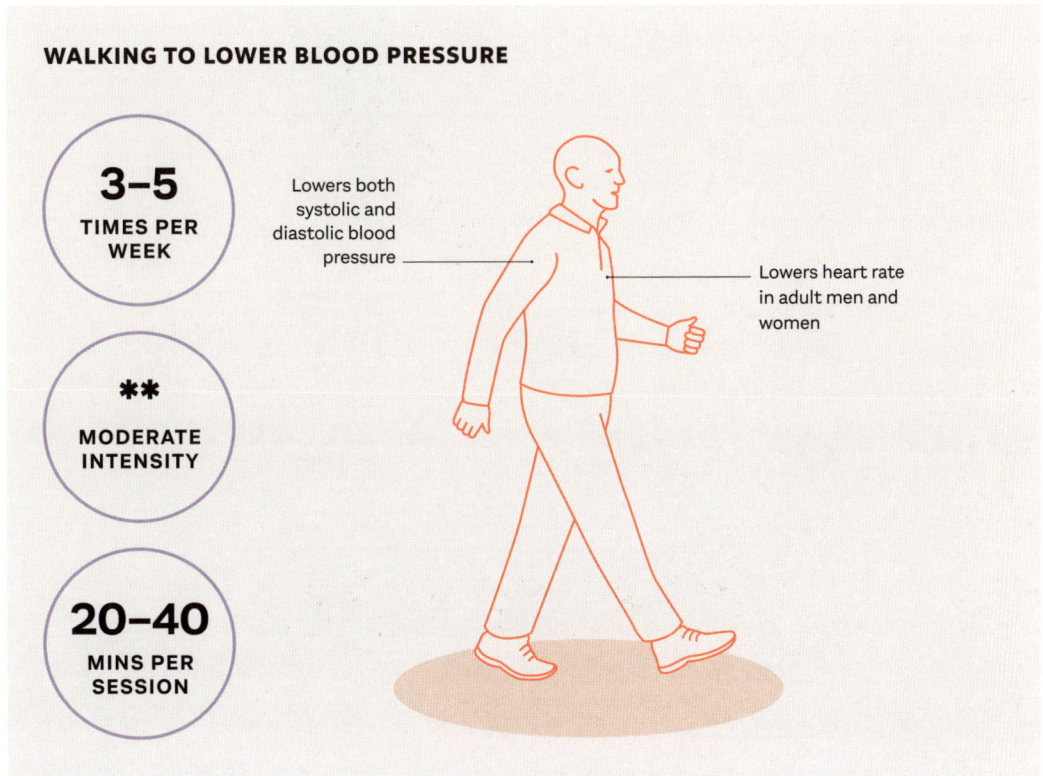

WALKING TO LOWER BLOOD PRESSURE

3–5 TIMES PER WEEK

** **MODERATE INTENSITY**

20–40 MINS PER SESSION

Lowers both systolic and diastolic blood pressure

Lowers heart rate in adult men and women

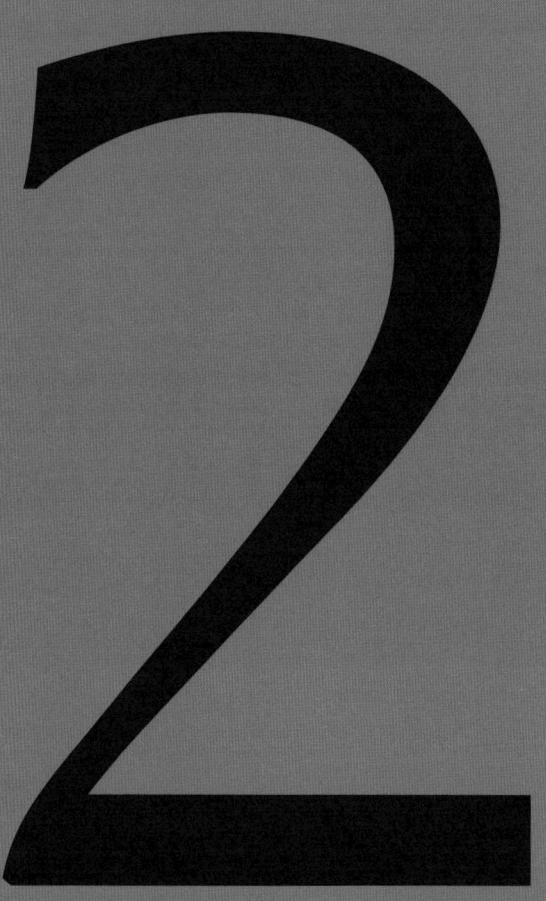

Getting started

Walking is the simplest form of activity, and your greatest investment will be a good pair of shoes, and your time. However, you will need to do some planning: What to wear? Where to go? For how long? With the right guidance and practical tips, you'll be ready to hit the road with confidence.

The right shoes for you

A good pair of shoes is the number-one item you will need in your walking toolkit. Looking after the biomechanics of your feet (bones, muscles, ligaments, and tendons) will help you to adopt good technique, prevent injuries, and allow you to walk in comfort for as long or as fast as you want.

Most feet fall into one of three walking styles: those that pronate, those that supinate, and those that are neutral. It is important that you know which category you fit into when you buy shoes, as some have insoles built in to correct excessive pronation or supination. To determine what kind of foot you have, try the following wet foot test.

ANALYSE YOUR FOOTPRINT
Dip your foot in water, shake off the excess, and then walk across a large sheet of card, or a dark-tiled floor if you have one. If you leave a footprint that forms a flat, solid band, with little or no distinction where the arch should be, then you are a **pronator**. A low arch, or flat feet, can exacerbate this. This is the most common bearing, and while a certain amount of pronation, where the foot rolls inwards and the arches flatten, is normal, with excessive pronation there is a marked inward roll of the foot as it lands. This can twist the foot, shin, knee, and hip, and stress the whole body. Another sign of pronation is rough skin forming on the inside edge of the foot and the heel.

If you leave a footprint that shows just the toes, ball of your foot, and heel, then you are a **supinator**. Supination is where the feet do not have enough inward motion, and roll to the outside edge of the foot after landing.

As a result, hard skin may form on the outside edge of the foot. If your footprint is somewhere in between the two, then your feet are **neutral**. Here, the foot neither excessively pronates nor supinates, and the centre of the heel strikes the ground. The soles of your shoes will also reveal more about your walking – study the diagrams opposite to learn more about tread wear.

CAUSES AND CURES
Excessive pronation and supination can be caused by corns, bunions, and other foot complaints, knee problems, or being overweight. Walking at even a few degrees out from the neutral gait can cause your body to overcompensate and take it out of alignment. For excessive pronation, find a shoe that will support the inside edge of your foot, with extra stability in the heel. Supinators should wear a shoe with good heel stability and extra cushioning under the ball of the foot. If you have a neutral gait, you can wear any good-quality shoe. You can self-treat minor pronation and, to a lesser degree, supination by using ready-made corrective insoles, or orthotics. These are designed to support your foot in the necessary places to correct your gait and prevent injury. However, if in doubt, seek advice from a qualified chiropodist or podiatrist and get a biomechanical assessment of your feet. A foot specialist will also arrange for bespoke orthotics to be made up for you.

KEY POINTS TO LOOK FOR

- Which is your bigger foot? It is common to have one foot bigger than the other. Buy shoes that fit your bigger foot, and make adjustments to the fit of the smaller foot with insoles.

- Are your feet wide or narrow? Many shoes come in one width, and while the fit can be adjusted slightly by the way that you lace your shoes (see pp42–43), if you have very wide or narrow feet you will need to buy shoes that are sold in different width sizes.

- Which is your longest toe? Usually, this is the big toe, but sometimes the second toe is the longest. There should be a two-finger width between the end of your longest toe and the end of the shoe.

- Do you have a slim heel? This is common for women, and may be combined with either a narrow or a wide fitting across the broadest part of the foot. Lacing your shoe to accommodate a narrow heel may help (see p43).

TREAD WEAR

The soles of an existing pair of your shoes will also reveal your walking gait. Place the heels together so that you can see them at eye level. If the heels are worn on the inside and the shoes lean in, then you pronate.

If the heels are worn on the outside and the shoes lean out, you supinate. If they are not excessively worn on either side, then your walking gait is neutral.

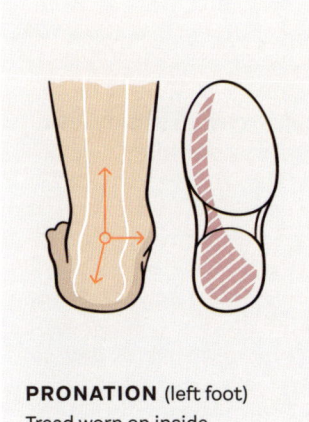

PRONATION (left foot)
Tread worn on inside

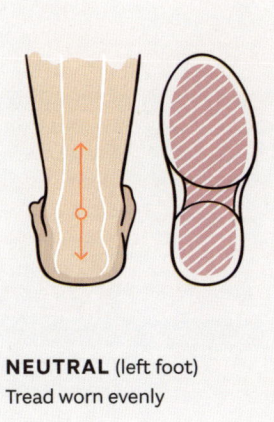

NEUTRAL (left foot)
Tread worn evenly

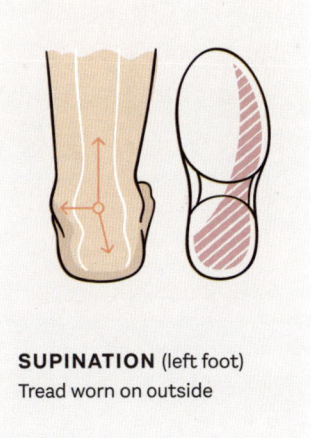

SUPINATION (left foot)
Tread worn on outside

SHOES FOR WALKING

Many people ask the question, "Can I wear a running shoe for walking?" Well, you wouldn't expect to perform well if you played tennis in football boots, and the same applies to walking and running shoes. A shoe suitable for walking must be flexible; at push off, a walker's forefoot flexes at nearly twice the angle of a runner's. The shoe needs to be pliable enough to follow the roll of the foot as you lead the heel-to-toe action. A walker lands on the heel, so good supportive cushioning in the heel is essential. The height of the heel on a walking shoe also needs to be on the low side. Many running shoes have quite a high heel profile, which when you walk can force you to overwork the shin muscles and cause injury.

It is important to find shoes that suit your feet. If you are unable to find a specific walking shoe, a cross trainer or a multi-terrain trail shoe is your next best choice. Aside from the key points (see pp40–41), a good starting place is to ensure the shoes are flexible, waterproof, and have good grip on the soles.

ORTHOTICS

These corrective insoles are designed to change the motion of the foot, in particular to relieve excessive pronation, and to stop further deterioration of the foot for those with flat feet or bunions. Preformed orthotics are available on the high street, while bespoke orthotics are made after a biomechanical assessment of your foot by a qualified podiatrist or chiropodist. They are designed specifically for your feet, and may include features such as heel lifts.

SHOPPING FOR SHOES

Choose a specialist athletics shoe shop that has a good reputation and trained staff. The staff should be able to assess your feet and direct you towards a selection of shoes that are right for you. The best shops have a treadmill so that you can try the shoes in action; some shops will even allow you to take a quick "test walk" outside on the pavement.

Buy shoes in the afternoon. Feet swell slightly throughout the day and when you walk vigorously, so always try on shoes when your feet are at their largest. Take with you a list of your foot dimensions (see pp36–37) so that you don't forget any important points about fit. Also make a note of any injuries past and present. They may have a bearing on which shoe you choose. Study pages 40-41 and note the key features you should be looking for in your walking shoes. Take your walking socks with you (see p49). You should always match these to your shoes so that they work together. Also take along your orthotics if you wear them. Finally, remember that shoes come in all price ranges, but expensive does not necessarily mean the best for you.

When you are trying on a pair of shoes, your feet should feel well supported and protected, comfortable and without any pressure on any part of your feet, held well in the heels, and supported under the arches. As with most sports shoes, walking shoes tend to be small for their size, and you will probably need to try on shoes that are between one and two sizes larger than you normally wear. Pay attention to the toe box. Some toe boxes can be quite tapered, and unless you have very slender feet your toes can bunch up slightly. This may feel fine in the shop, but as soon as you start to walk any distance your toes will start to rub against the shoe, causing blisters and bruising. Make sure, too, that there is a two-finger width between your longest toe and the end of your shoe.

You should not have to "wear in" shoes. If they pinch or rub in the slightest way, leave them on the shelf. You want to walk out of the shop ready to go a million miles.

CARING FOR YOUR SHOES

Now that you have the perfect shoes, help them to last. If you get your shoes wet, remove the insoles and dry them separately. Stuff the shoes with newspaper to absorb the moisture, and dry them slowly away from direct heat. Remove the paper after a few hours once it has soaked up as much moisture as possible. Don't try to hurry the drying process by putting wet shoes on or near a heat source, such as radiator, as this will make the materials in the shoe crack and weaken. Do not put your shoes in the washing machine to clean them. Again, this will speed the breakdown of materials in the shoe. Wipe off any dirt with a damp cloth and leave them to air. If your shoes are very muddy, lightly scrub off the mud under lukewarm running water. Then dry them as before. Don't store your shoes in a plastic bag or box. Leave them out to air between wearings. If possible, buy two pairs of shoes so that you can rotate their use.

FOR HIKING ONLY

The features of a rigid sole and ankle support that make hiking boots ideal for taking you across very soft or rugged terrain can cause severe damage to your feet if worn for walking long distances on tarmac, or any kind of fast walking. Always wear the right shoes!

Replace your shoes every 800–1125km (500–700 miles); write the date of purchase inside the shoe so you don't forget. After this amount of wear they may still look good on the outside, but they will have deteriorated on the inside to the point where they no longer support your foot properly. My shoes usually let me know when they need changing. A really comfortable pair of shoes will suddenly start to give me blisters, or pain in my ankles, as the support slackens.

"You should not have to 'wear in' shoes. If they pinch or rub in the slightest way, leave them on the shelf. You want to walk out of the shop ready to go a million miles."

WHAT TO LOOK FOR

A shoe suitable for walking must ideally be light and flexible so that it can mimic the range of movement from the foot. Whether you plan on walking a few miles a day, taking on a marathon, or hiking a distance, the key principles of choosing your footwear are the same. Check that the toe box is roomy and rounded so that your toes can move freely; unless you have very slender feet, avoid tapered toe boxes. You will need to have at least a two-finger width between your longest toe and the end of the shoe to allow sufficient space for the push-off movement. Finally, always make sure your chosen socks work with your shoes!

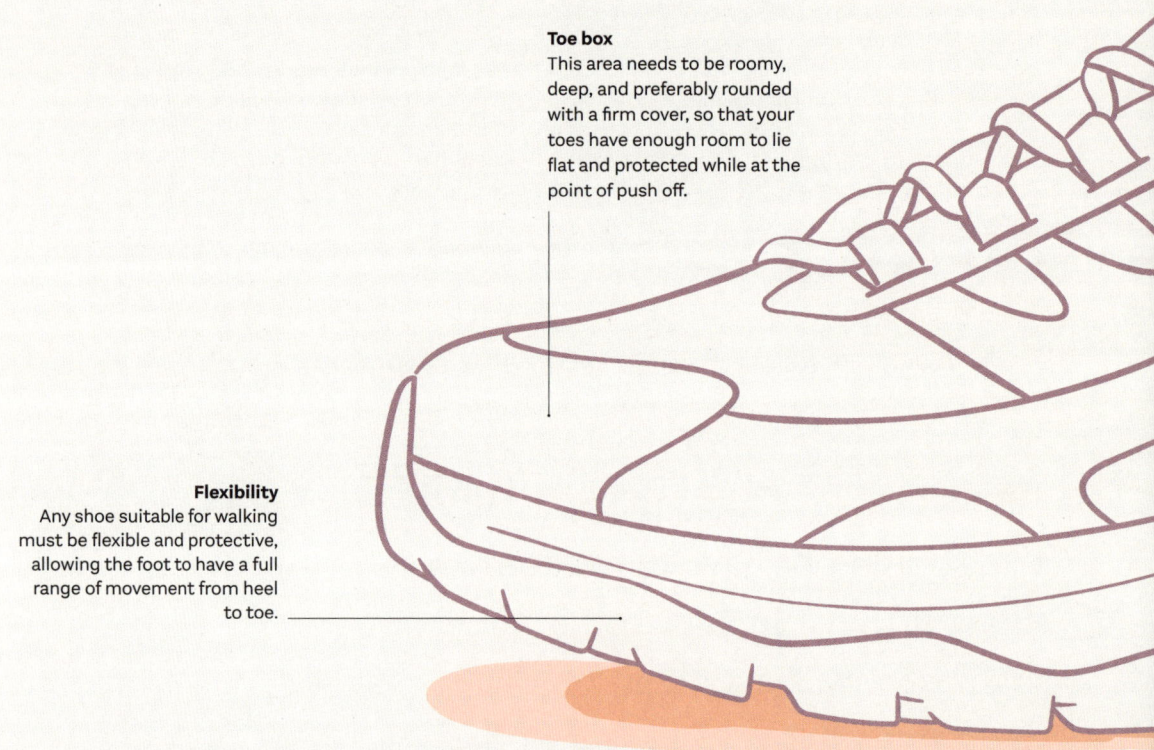

Toe box
This area needs to be roomy, deep, and preferably rounded with a firm cover, so that your toes have enough room to lie flat and protected while at the point of push off.

Flexibility
Any shoe suitable for walking must be flexible and protective, allowing the foot to have a full range of movement from heel to toe.

Low cut heel
Due to the acute angle of the ankle every time you push off, a low heel profile will help prevent pressing against the Achilles tendon and any risk of injuring this very fragile part of the foot.

Lightweight and waterproof
A good walking shoe should be as light and flexible as possible. For some conditions, choose a waterproof shoe made from a Gore-Tex material.

Cushioning
Supportive cushioning is essential, especially in the heel and under the ball of the foot.

Arch support
In any good walking shoe there should be an effective arch support and insole.

Stability
If you pronate or supinate, look for a heel that will support and correct this. Or for some, as it does not suit everyone, look into a zero drop where the entire foot is on the same level.

GETTING STARTED 41

LACING TECHNIQUES

The way that you lace your shoes can further improve the fit. This is especially useful if, for example, you have a wide foot but a narrow heel.

Always loosen your laces before you slip into the shoes to prevent stress on the eyelets and wear on the heels. Tighten your laces from the bottom eyelets, closest to your toes, to the top of the shoe, pulling the laces tight at each set of eyelets before going on to the next set.

LACING FOR A WIDE FOOT

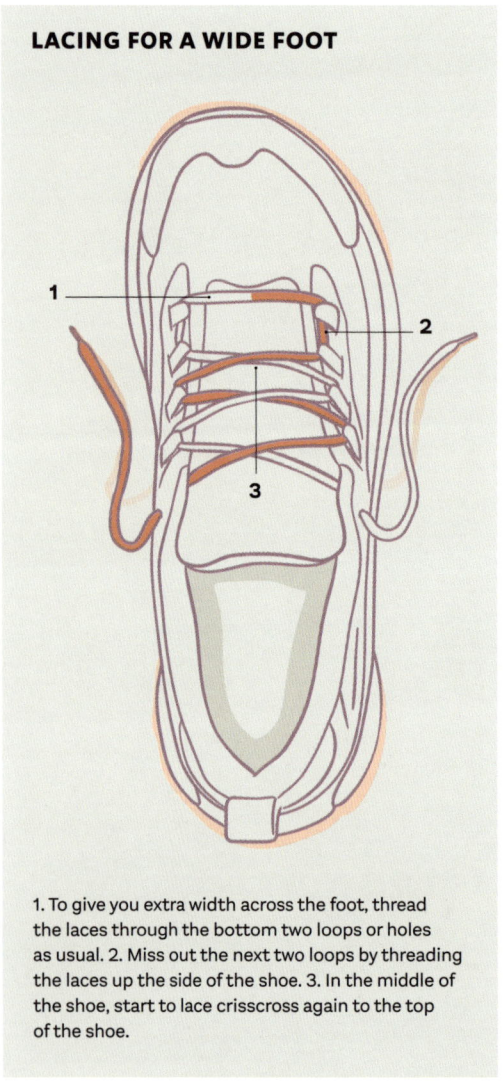

1. To give you extra width across the foot, thread the laces through the bottom two loops or holes as usual. 2. Miss out the next two loops by threading the laces up the side of the shoe. 3. In the middle of the shoe, start to lace crisscross again to the top of the shoe.

LACING FOR A NARROW FOOT

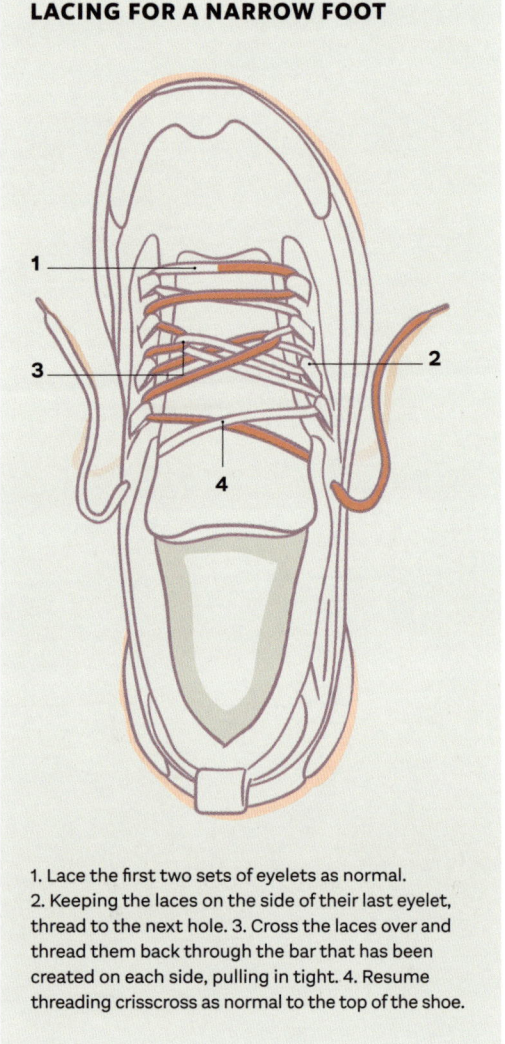

1. Lace the first two sets of eyelets as normal. 2. Keeping the laces on the side of their last eyelet, thread to the next hole. 3. Cross the laces over and thread them back through the bar that has been created on each side, pulling in tight. 4. Resume threading crisscross as normal to the top of the shoe.

The standard crisscross lacing suits most people, and allows you to tighten the laces more evenly than bar lacing. Most shoes have double eyelets at the top. Use them both for a firm fit for a slim foot, or leave the top set unlaced if you have a high instep or a broad foot.

LACING FOR A WIDE OR DEEP ARCH

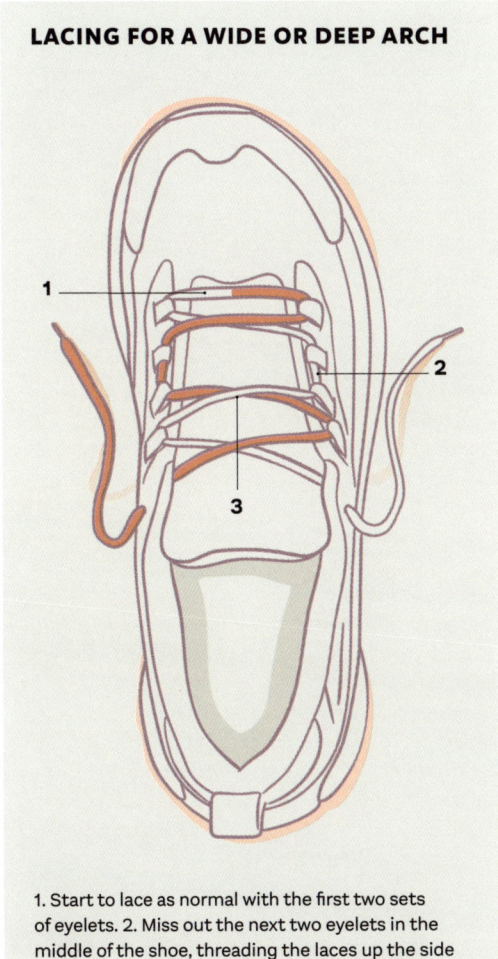

1. Start to lace as normal with the first two sets of eyelets. 2. Miss out the next two eyelets in the middle of the shoe, threading the laces up the side of the shoe. 3. Continue lacing as normal to the top of the shoe.

LACING FOR A NARROW OR SLIPPING HEEL

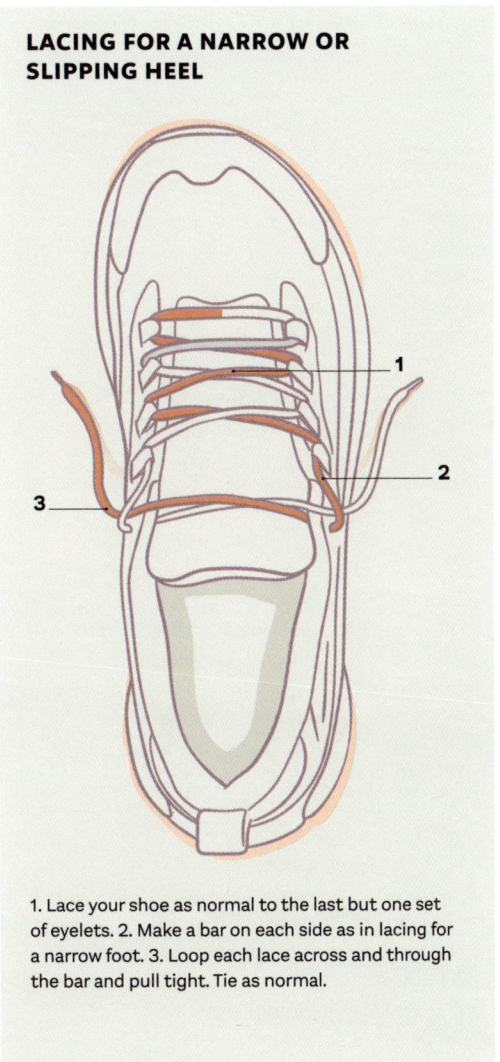

1. Lace your shoe as normal to the last but one set of eyelets. 2. Make a bar on each side as in lacing for a narrow foot. 3. Loop each lace across and through the bar and pull tight. Tie as normal.

Injuries

As a low impact activity, walking is unlikely to be the cause of injury, although it can exacerbate past injuries, so it's always good to get checked before embarking on any goal if it is above and beyond your usual walking activity. Poorly fitting shoes can also be the root cause for some common problems; see pp36–37 for advice on choosing the right shoes.

BLISTERS

Causes and symptoms Blisters are caused by continual rubbing against the skin. A bubble of fluid forms, pocketed between the top layers of skin, and when pressure is applied it feels painful. Poorly fitting shoes are a common cause of blisters. Socks that are too big, too small, or too old and worn can also result in blisters. Other causes are rough skin or wet feet, either from extreme sweating or walking in rain.

Treatment and prevention The standard advice is to let the fluid subside naturally and if this hasn't happened after 24 hours, to lance the bubble to drain the fluid. I find blisters don't heal quickly unless you lance the bubble immediately. You can sterilize the needle with antiseptic wash, in boiling water, or by heating it in a flame. Pierce two little holes, at either end of the blister. Using sterile gauze, press down gently to remove the liquid.

Wipe the area with an antiseptic solution, and then cover with non-allergenic dressing tape, not lint. This will form a replacement for the skin, allowing the blister to heal in half the time. If blisters repeatedly return in the same place, check the size and width fitting of your shoes to make sure they are compatible with your feet (see p38). If you suspect your socks are the problem, try a different sort (see p49). Try covering your feet in petroleum jelly or blister powders that you shake into your shoes. These act as a barrier and protect the feet from being rubbed. Prevention is better than cure, so taping any areas that can become hot spots before you set off, can make a big difference.

ATHLETE'S FOOT

Causes and symptoms This is a fungus that appears between the toes and on the soles of the feet as cracks of red, flaky, itchy skin that can be quite painful. It can cross-infect from foot-to-nail or nail-to-foot.

Treatment and prevention Apply an anti-fungal (fungicide) cream to the infected areas as directed on the packaging. There are many products available. If athlete's foot returns, as it often does, treat it with a different brand of cream as the fungus may form a tolerance to your usual brand. Continue treating the area for two weeks after the symptoms have disappeared because the fungus can still remain up to this point.

To help prevent a return of the fungus, keep your feet clean and dry at all times. Wear socks made of synthetic fabrics that will wick the moisture from your skin. It is important to also treat your shoes and socks, because washing them is not enough to destroy the fungus.

BLACK TOENAILS

Causes and symptoms Black toenails are usually caused by shoes that are too small. Each time you push off from your toes as you walk, the toes bang against the end of the toe box in the shoe. Over time this bruises the toes and causes a pooling of blood under the nail, which then blackens. The toe will be painful and will throb under the pressure of the blood that has collected.

Treatment and prevention you can preserve your toenail by puncturing it with a sterilized needle through the nail. This is painless, but must be done within an hour of the black toenail appearing. If you don't catch it early enough, or if it isn't too painful, leave it to heal naturally. The nail will fall off after a few months, and new nail will have grown underneath. Make sure there is a two finger width between the end of your longest toe to the top of the shoe, and wear thicker socks to cushion your toes.

INGROWN TOENAILS

Causes and symptoms Ingrown nails occur mostly on the big toe and may be caused by poorly fitting shoes. How you cut and file your toenails may also encourage the toenail to grow into the skin, especially if the toenail is curved or has been cut too short on the sides of the nail. They can be very painful, particularly when the shoe adds pressure to the nail. The skin around the nail will appear red and inflamed, and may become infected.

Treatment and prevention Soak the affected foot in a bowl of warm water to which you have added 2–4 drops of tea tree essential oil or 1–2 tablespoons of salt at least once a day. If you are unable to cut the nail because it has become embedded in the skin, see a chiropodist, podiatrist, or your doctor. Always cut toenails straight across, making sure you file any sharp corners with an emery board.

PLANTAR FASCIITIS

Causes and symptoms This is an inflammation of the plantar fascia, a band of thick tissue that binds the muscle in the sole of the foot, caused by too much stress being placed on the area. It is easy to detect because the pain in your heel will be felt immediately as you get up in the morning or after sitting for some time and then lessens as the day goes on. The pain is often described as feeling like a "bone bruise". Common causes are continually standing, being overweight, having flat feet (especially if they overpronate, see p36), high arched feet, worn-out shoes which allow overpronation, or a tightness in the Achilles tendon.

Treatment and prevention Apply an ice pack to the area for 15–20 minutes four times a day and elevate the foot whenever possible. Healing cannot be rushed, and can take weeks if not months, so you may have to be patient. If you still feel pain after prolonged treatment, visit a chiropodist. You may need heel cups and padding or orthotics (see p38) to treat the real problem rather than the symptoms. Roll a small ball underneath your foot, pressing down to get the depth of massage you require. Work on stretching and strengthening the Achilles tendon and calf muscles (see p87 and p93). Check that your shoes are not too worn and support your arches (see p36 and p38).

SWOLLEN FINGERS

Causes and symptoms Fingers swell and become cold when the blood supply is depleted. This can happen when your arms and hands are down at your sides while walking.

Treatment and prevention Keep your arms at a 90-degree angle and regularly clench and unclench your fists. By using the correct arm movement, you encourage good blood flow. Wearing gloves also makes a big difference.

What to wear

Following shoes, your next big decision is what to wear when walking. Key considerations are comfort, practicality, and safety, along with when, where, and how far you intend to go. The goal is that you feel well equipped and prepared from head to toe so that all your attention can be on enjoying your walk!

CHOOSE YOUR LAYERS

I would never suggest spending a lot of money on a walking kit, but it can be miserable if it doesn't do the job. For your legs, opt for leggings or shorts that will not get wet and flap around your ankles. Make sure any legwear is loose enough around the waist, and made of a fabric, like polyester, that will wick any moisture away from your body. Due to the scissor-like action of your legs while walking, avoid jogging pants, jeans, or any trousers with raised inside seams as they can cause chafing and discomfort on the inside of your thighs.

A common mistake that people make when starting to walk regularly is wearing too many clothes. Your body temperature can rise and fall quite dramatically depending on the speed or intensity of your walk. The trick is to begin by wearing three different layers, choosing technical clothing with moisture-wicking fabrics that will keep you dry, warm, or cool.

Base layer Ideally a thin, long- or short-sleeved layer. Choose either a technical T-shirt, or a Merino wool layer; both will help to keep you dry. While a cotton T-shirt feels lovely to put on, once wet with sweat it is hard to get dry, and feels cold to wear.

Mid layer The thickness should be based on where you are walking. A polar fleece or a Merino layer is lightweight, and can be bought in seasonal thicknesses for varying degrees of warmth. They can easily pack down into a small backpack or tie around the waist when not being worn and both are extremely breathable. Always have a layer to put on at the end of your walk.

Outer layer This is your lightweight windbreaker and waterproof layer, intended to keep you dry on the outside, but allowing your body to breathe and expel moisture from the inside. Depending on your demands, check the technical specification for its rating and other features that you may need. Hiking trousers can also be made of the same fabric and are even more useful if they come with zip-off legs so that they can convert into shorts. Where possible wear bright high visibility colours and clothing that has reflective strips so that from dawn to dusk and in the dark, you can easily be seen. See page 54 for more on walking safety.

HIGH-PERFORMANCE WEAR

The science of fitness clothing has come a long way, and while the beauty of walking is that you do not have to have specific clothing, being prepared and selective about what you wear, so that you stay comfortable and dry in all weathers, can determine how much you enjoy your walk.

Head protection
An ear warmer, or preferably a hat, retains heat in winter. A baseball cap is ideal for protection from the sun and keeping rain off your face in wet weather. Avoid cotton and choose a technical wicking fabric.

High-visibility reflective clothing
For your own safety, be seen at all times, especially at night or in poor weather conditions.

Vest or T-shirt
The aim is to stay cool in the heat and warm when it's cold. A high-wicking top that will not absorb sweat makes an excellent base garment, which you can then add layers over as necessary.

Gloves
Necessary for the cooler months, choose gloves with touch screen compatible fingertips. This will enable you to look at any GPS device without having to remove them.

Long-sleeved layer
A light, long-sleeved breathable garment that is also water repellent can provide a layer of warmth when needed. Ensure that the sleeves are loose enough to swing your arms, and if possible have underarm or side zips that can be opened, allowing air to circulate when required.

Bum bag
The ideal bum bag should be able to hold all the items you may need, but be compact enough not to interfere with your walking technique.

Water holder
Using a water holder will allow you to carry up to 750ml (1¼ pints), leaving you completely free to focus on your arm movements.

Leggings or shorts
These should have good stretch and fit comfortably with no raised inside seams that can rub.

A GOOD FOUNDATION

It is estimated that 70 per cent of women are wearing the wrong size bra, and for sports bras, possibly higher. Regardless of cup size, it is important to have a bra fitting prior to buying any sports bra, making sure it is the correct size, and offers the necessary support for the level of activity planned. The breasts are made of delicate tissue, not muscle. Vigorous movement may stretch or tear the tissue, and once it has been damaged, the tissue cannot repair itself, so having the necessary support is essential.

It is worth bearing in mind that regular exercise will almost definitely change your body shape over a period of time, and your bra size may change, too. Most sports bras now come with information as to the level and type of exercise they are most suited for. Walking can easily range from moderate to vigorous, depending on your goal. A sports bra is designed to hold your breasts close to you so there is minimal movement. Because they can feel tighter than a normal bra, it is important that they have moisture-wicking properties to allow your skin to breathe.

Some bras include a silver fibre, which is said to neutralize bacteria in the area. Others are designed to house a heart-rate monitor, a useful feature if you want to wear one. Buy two sports bras so that having one in the wash does not stop you walking. Replace a sports bra

SPORTS BRAS

A well-fitting sports bra should feel snug, but not so tight that it affects your breathing. Look for broad, non-elastic straps that won't cut into your shoulders. Padded straps will give extra comfort. Make sure that the underband of the bra fits firmly around the ribcage so that it doesn't move when you are walking or reaching up.

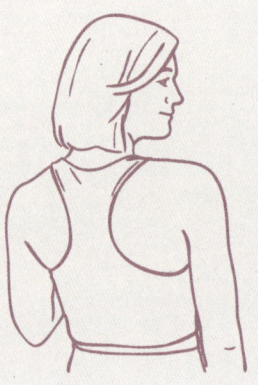

High impact support
Sports bras with moulded cups that encapsulate each breast give firmer support, and are ideal for women with fuller breasts. Avoid sports bras that hook together at the front, as these tend to allow more breast motion. Look for pull-on types, or ones that hook at the back. The "Y-back" panel gives good support, and the open design allows a greater area of skin to breathe freely.

Moderate impact support
Cropped-top bras can be worn as outerwear and have compressed cups fitted inside. These flatten the breasts against the body, keeping breast motion to a minimum, and are most suitable for women with smaller breasts. Cropped-top bras often have reflective strips on them so you can be seen in the dark. The "Y-back" panel on the back gives good support for all sizes.

within 6–12 months, especially if you are walking 3–4 times a week. Over time, it will lose its elasticity and start to feel loose, which is a clear sign that it needs replacing.

SOCKS

Some people swear by thin socks, but personally, I prefer a thicker sock with padding in the sensitive areas, under the ball of the foot, around the toes, and over the Achilles. Toe socks also offer another alternative. Whichever type of sock you choose, stick to synthetic fibres that will wick away moisture and dry quickly; cotton or wool socks, unless they are smart wool, can cause blisters when they get wet. Make sure that your socks are a good fit, not too tight and restricting, and reach high enough to cover your Achilles tendon. Replace your socks as soon as you can see that they are wearing thin on the heels or elsewhere. Never wear your shoes without socks.

Which sock to choose?

There are so many styles of sports socks to choose from so it is trial and error until you find the right one for you. Good walking socks can cost more, but are worth the investment. Nothing beats wearing a great pair of socks in the right-fitting shoes. Always choose synthetic fibres over natural ones; they are better at drawing moisture away from your skin.

Thick socks with extra padding These are my favourite type of socks. They feel soft and luxurious, and have extra padded areas at strategic points on the foot, in the ball and heel, and sometimes over the arch of the foot, too. Wear your thick socks when buying shoes as they can make up to half a size difference.

Thin socks Look for minimal or no seams and avoid cotton – check they are made from synthetic materials. They do not offer much protection, but it is a personal choice.

Double-layer socks These are made with two layers of fabric and are designed to prevent blisters. The theory is that as you move, the two layers rub against each other rather than against your foot. I feel that they are more successful for runners than for walkers.

Toe socks These separate the toes to eliminate skin-on-skin friction. They can also help to improve balance and movement. Make sure they are a good fit with your shoes.

Low-cut ankle socks These are not recommended, as your Achilles tendon continually hits the back of your shoes.

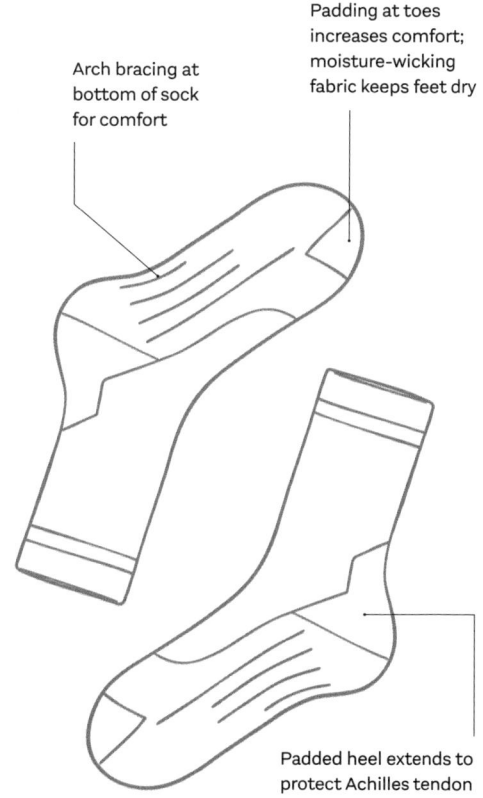

Arch bracing at bottom of sock for comfort

Padding at toes increases comfort; moisture-wicking fabric keeps feet dry

Padded heel extends to protect Achilles tendon

Walking in different climates

Rarely are the weather conditions so bad that they prevent you from enjoying your walk. Walking on crisp new snow or with the sun on your skin can be a great experience. When walking in extreme heat or cold, prepare by wearing the correct clothing, knowing your limitations, and being aware of what you need to do to make yourself safe and comfortable.

Always check the weather forecast so that you can decide if a walk is possible that day and prepare for the conditions. Even the fittest person will have days when a walk is out of the question. Note that temperatures above 35°C (95°F) or below -23°C (-10°F) are always unsafe.

When walking in extreme heat, be cautious and slow your pace down if the temperature is above 26°C (80°F). Also check the humidity level. High humidity can push the apparent temperature up to 5°C (41°F) because the moisture in the air prevents your sweat from evaporating, and it is the evaporation that cools you. Heat stroke and heat exhaustion can be very serious. To avoid suffering from either, walk at the coolest times of day, before 11.00am and after 3.00pm. You may need to slow your pace and keep alert to how you feel. At the first sign of dizziness or a headache, stop walking, find shade, and cool down.

TIPS ON KEEPING COOL

- Freeze half a bottle of water and top it up with cold water before you set out. You will then have a cool drink, at least until the ice melts.

- To lower your temperature, soak a cooling towel in cold water and then wrap around your neck or head to help evaporate your sweat.

- Listen to your body, slow your pace, and wear light, wicking clothing that does not expose your skin to the sun.

TIPS ON KEEPING WARM

- Alter your stride so that your pace is shorter and quicker to raise the heart rate and keep you warm.

- Always wear a hat that covers your ears – 60 per cent of your body heat is lost through the top of the head.

- Carry a small, hand-held hot pack to warm your hands if you really feel the chill.

- If you have asthma you may want to breathe warm air, so wear a scarf to cover your chin and mouth.

KEEPING COOL IN THE HEAT

When walking in heat, always carry and drink plenty of water to stay hydrated. Your body will sweat more than in normal weather, and can need as much as double your normal intake of water to replace lost fluids. Drink 0.6 litres (1 pint) of water both before and after your walk and drink regularly during, at least every 15–20 minutes. While preoccupied with walking, you may be unaware of the sun's intensity until it is too late.

Wear light or white clothes to reflect the sun's heat, and choose those that are made from very light moisture-wicking fabrics. Invest in sun-protective clothing if you can; their sun protection factor (SPF) ranges from SPF 30 to SPF 100. Wear clothing that covers the body rather than exposing it. A hat is essential, preferably one that covers the back of your neck, and you should always wear UV protection sunglasses. Apply a suitable strength sun cream liberally all over, even under your clothes, then re-apply later, because sweating will rub it off.

PROTECTING AGAINST THE COLD

In cold conditions it is essential to warm up and stretch thoroughly before setting out. Do your cooldown stretches indoors, and after your walk, if you have been sweating, change out of your clothes quickly to avoid feeling chilled.

Be aware of the wind chill factor, which can turn a cold day into a freezing one. In cold conditions your heart has to work extra hard for you to walk and keep warm. If you have a heart problem, you should consult a doctor before walking in very cold weather. To avoid the most severe conditions, try to walk in the middle, and warmest, part of the day.

Wear layers that you can take off if you get too warm. Begin with a thermal smart wool base layer, followed by a mid-layer fleece. Choose a three- to four-season hard shell jacket that is lightweight, breathable, packable, and offers good all-round weather protection. Check it has a high waterproof specification (see box below). For added warmth, wear thermal longjohns under your leggings or trousers, but nothing to restrict movement. A Gore-Tex shoe or boot is ideal for keeping your feet dry, but beware, if you suffer from hot sweaty feet they can also trap moisture in.

OUT IN THE RAIN OR WIND

- For wind and rain you need a jacket that has a high breathability rating of over 10,000g/mm, which is ideal for moderate activity, or up to 20,000g/mm for more aerobic activity and intense hiking. This is not the same as having just a waterproofing which, as soon as you are active, will turn the jacket into a sauna.

- Make sure that the jacket cuffs can be drawn tight to keep water out, and that the back is long enough to cover your bottom and keep it dry. The neck of the jacket should be high enough to keep out drips, and a peaked hood, whether a simple fold-away or zip-off version, will stop rain from falling on your face.

- For a layer of warmth without adding bulk, you may want to wear weather-resistant gloves. From fleece to Merino wool there is a wide choice available.

- For walking in strong winds, you need a jacket with a drawstring bottom to keep the wind out.

Walking technology and accessories

One of the many benefits of walking is that you do not need specialist equipment. As long as you have on a good pair of shoes, you can open your front door and go. However, tracking your walking and training progress can be really helpful and very motivating. Technology is there to help, literally every step of the way.

PEDOMETERS, GPS, AND SMARTPHONES

Measuring distances has never been easier. You can now choose from an overwhelming number of devices that can measure anything and everything, either on a specific device or by apps downloaded onto your smartphone. It is all at your fingertips.

A small pedometer or pedometer bracelet is the most basic and low cost option and ideal for beginners. These will track key information such as distance, pace, step count, and time. Plus, some will also have a calorie counter so that you can check on energy used during your walk.

Moving up a notch, there are devices designed to be worn 24 hours a day. These will do all of the above, plus keep track of your steps and calories used each day, record your heart rate, track your sleep patterns, and also play music. A smart watch will give alerts via texts and emails, as well as many other features that can support not only your health and fitness, but also your daily life.

Your smartphone can make the perfect training partner. The downside is that in certain areas the GPS signal can be unreliable. It is also important to be aware that from a safety perspective they can be distracting.

APPS

There are a number of apps that you can download to support your walking goals, including individual apps to measure distance, pace, predict calories used, tell you what to eat, measure your heart rate, monitor your sleeping, or just to motivate you to the next challenge. Depending on the range of support you are looking for, choose apps that combine different features so that you don't have to juggle multiple apps.

When choosing the app that you need, be selective as to the quality and the information it will provide. Check to see if it is set by gender, or if it requires personal information as well as setting your goals and fitness ambitions.

The data from your device can be transferred to your app so that you have an instant walking log that will keep track of your week in, week out progress.

HOW TO FIT IT ALL TOGETHER

Start by wearing the device every day for one week. Put it on in the morning and wear it until bedtime. Some people may decide to wear it at night to monitor sleep patterns. By the end of the week you will have information on your average daily steps, which may really surprise you! It is important to note that the number of steps taken throughout the day should be in addition to any mileage that you complete on a training plan. However, depending on your level of fitness, you may need to gently build up the distances.

WALK BAGS FOR ESSENTIALS

A bum bag is a really useful bit of kit, regardless of the distance you intend to walk. You can keep it loaded with all the essentials that you might need. Use it to carry a few first, aid items, keys, money, lip salve, sunglasses, and your phone (see also p55).

For comfort, make sure that the bag fits into the small of your back to avoid it bouncing up and down as you walk. Ideally it should come with a water bottle holder either attached, or as a separate unit.

If you really do not like to feel anything around your waist, use a wrist or arm pouch. This is a small zipped purse, just big enough to take keys and money, that has a Velcro strap to fit it snugly around the arm. You can also find arm pouches to hold your phone or device.

Avoid backpacks – they are bad for your posture and even the lightweight packs will tend to cut into your shoulders after a few miles. However, if you are hiking on trails (see pp126–127) you may want to invest in a light backpack with well-padded straps.

HEART-RATE MONITORS

For most everyday users a heart-rate monitor worn on the wrist as part of a smart watch will be more than adequate, taking into account gender, age, height, and body weight, etc.
If you need a more accurate reading, either for a health condition or a specific challenge, it is better to wear a chest strap monitor.

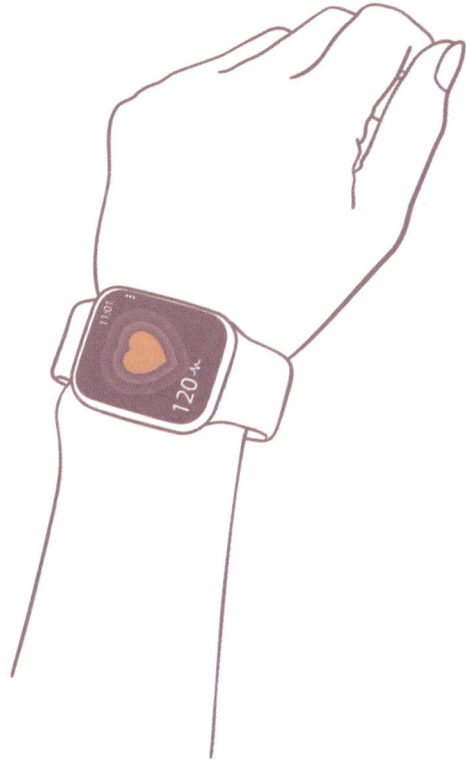

GETTING STARTED

Safety

Whether you are walking in a busy city, or on a quiet country lane, alone or with a group, it is important that you know how to walk safely. By using your common sense combined with some practical advice, you should feel confident and well prepared for any walk.

The secret of walking safely is forward planning.

Step one: Make sure you keep a ready-packed bum bag or a small day backpack with all the essential items, and use a water bottle holder.

Step two: Plan your route carefully.

Step three: Wear high-visibility clothing with reflective strips both on your front and back. It doesn't matter what time of day you are walking or the weather conditions; it is important to be seen at all times.

Step four: Ensure you have a fully charged phone, and on longer walks take a portable charger. Make sure you have installed the ICE app (in case of emergency). This will place any important medical information or contact details visibly onto the screen of a locked phone. Or, you can write the information in permanent ink on the inside flap of your bum bag. Following these simple guidelines will allow you to feel more relaxed and in control.

WALK BAG ESSENTIALS

The following list may seem like a lot of items, but it is better to be prepared for any eventuality. Choose a bum bag or a light day bag that is compact, and ideally with several pockets so that you can find things easily. Keep a small pot of petroleum jelly to rub onto your feet in case your shoes begin to rub, and for your lips, especially in cold weather. Tissues, surgical tape for any blister-prone areas, and a few adhesive bandages are good to have for any minor injuries. Good old paper and a short pencil can be useful for making any notes that come to mind. (I always have my most creative thoughts while walking!)

Carry a card, have access to cards on your phone, or carry enough money to buy extra water and snacks, as well as to cover the cost of a taxi or transportation home if required. Add your local taxi company to your phone contacts. You may want to include a pollution mask if you regularly walk in areas of heavy traffic and want to cut down on inhaling exhaust fumes. Carrying a small personal alarm that you know how to use, a phone charger, and a head torch can be useful, especially if you plan to be walking at night or out for some time. Always keep your bag loaded and ready to go so that each time you walk, you only need to remember water, keys, phone, and something to snack on (such as a banana or cereal bar).

PLAN YOUR ROUTE

There are plenty of apps you can use to plot and plan a variety of routes, which will also fit in with any fitness or walking plan you may be using. When you have determined your route, always check it in daylight and by car before setting off on foot. For safety and maintaining interest, it is always a good idea to regularly change your route.

WALKING IN THE DARK

It is not enough just to wear light-coloured clothes when walking at night, or when visibility is poor. High-visibility clothing helps you to be seen and recognized as a moving body. Most shoes and technical sports clothing come with reflective marks, but you can also buy separate accessories for added safety. Carry a head torch in case you need additional light. At night choose walks that are preferably in well-lit areas. It can be lovely to walk alone, but always let somebody know where you are walking and what time you expect to return. If it is really unavoidable that your walk travels through areas you are unsure of, it is better to walk with a friend. The limited daylight hours of winter walking can be challenging, so creating your own walking group can be a good option.

SAFETY CHECK LIST

☑ Carry a loaded bum bag with all your essentials, plus a holder for your water so that your hands are kept free.

☑ Fully charge your phone and add ICE (in case of emergency) details. Avoid using your phone to chat, or using any other electronic devices that take your attention off the road while walking. Be aware of your environment – be it a dog, cyclist, a fast car, or other people around you.

☑ Always walk in the direction facing the oncoming traffic if your route does not have pavements or bike paths. Try to avoid any areas that you are unsure of.

☑ Dress to be seen and wear reflective clothing. Drivers are not expecting to see you. At the very least, wear a white T shirt over your training kit.

☑ Carrying a personal alarm can make you feel more comfortable and make sure you know how to use it.

☑ Always trust your instincts. If you feel uneasy at any time, breathe out slowly to help you relax and gain control. Keep moving and head for a busy area to ask for help in a shop or café.

☑ Always try to look confident and aware of your surroundings. When walking towards a stranger, keep your eyes neutral. Allow your gaze to rest briefly on the person, then look to either side of them. This signals that you are not fazed by his or her presence.

☑ Carry the number of a local taxi company and a card or enough money for transport home should you need it.

☑ Enjoy planning and trying out new routes in daylight, preferably by car before starting to walk them. Allow others to track your location while you walk.

☑ Avoid unnecessary risk and prepare. Before venturing out, ask yourself, "Who am I walking with?", "Where will I, or we, walk?", "Does somebody know where I am walking?", "Do I have everything I need?", "Do I have enough water?", "Is my phone fully charged?" Most importantly, use your common sense and awareness to continually re-evaluate your surroundings while you are walking.

Planning your route

Great pleasure can be found in spontaneously choosing to go for a walk, but it can also be frustrating. It can be difficult to judge the distance, which means sometimes a walk can be over too soon, or that you have to go further than you had intended. The key is to establish your walking ability, then map out a range of routes that match your level of fitness.

Whatever your fitness level in other activities, if you are new to walking you need to discover your ability before you plan any routes. The best way to do this is to walk 1.6km (1 mile), or whatever distance suits you, and record how long it took you and how you felt on finishing.

MEASURE YOUR ABILITY

The ideal place to test your speed and ability over a controlled distance is on a running or athletics track, usually found in schools or parks. You may need to ask permission to use one. As a general rule, the inside lane of a standard track has a distance of 402 metres (440 yards), but they do vary, so always check the length. To walk 1.6km (1 mile) you will need to walk round the inside track four times. As you move outwards from the inside lane, each track increases in length by about 7 metres (7.5 yards). A track is useful when measuring your ability because there is no traffic, plus you will find toilet facilities and access to water. It is also a safe place to stop if you feel uncomfortable at any time. The other option is to measure the distance of 1.6km (1 mile) by car or by bike on a road, for you to walk afterwards. Try to make it a circular route so that you are never far from home, just in case you need to stop. Walk at your fastest pace, but without straining yourself, and time how long this set distance takes you (remember to warm up and cool down, see p90). It may take 15 minutes, it may take 30 minutes or more, or perhaps you will need to stop before the end. When you have finished, assess your progress. For example, could you have carried on walking? Did your legs ache? Was it a struggle, and were you out of breath? The answers to these questions will help you to decide your next move. If you are able to walk 1.6km (1 mile) easily, you are ready to begin one of the programmes (see pp144-181). When you start your programme, listen to your body, and if the regime feels too easy or too hard, try another one at a different level. Revisit this test after a few weeks to monitor your progress.

If you struggled to complete the course, you will probably want to walk at your own pace and distance for a few weeks to become accustomed to the exercise. For example, try just one lap of the track, or points on your route for either 0.4km or 0.8km (¼ or ½ mile). See if you can reach either of these markers, and build up from there.

FINDING FAVOURITE ROUTES

Having established your walking ability, and the distance of your first walk, you need to research two or three routes. Some walks will be more successful than others, and it is trial and error to build up a list of your favourite routes. Be realistic – if a route takes too much organization, or if you are unsure of the area, then you simply won't walk it. It is important that you enjoy the surroundings. Accessibility, variety, and enjoyment should be your guides when planning walks.

URBAN WALKING

There are many benefits of city walking: there is plenty of tarmac and pavement to achieve a constant stride pattern, and you can find a variety of routes, from city streets and colourful markets to parks, canal paths, or even historic landmarks. Research your area and plot routes that explore your local surroundings.

"Mall Walking", which is hugely popular in the US, is another option. It provides a safe, climate-controlled environment, long corridors offering a variety of routes and distances, and facilities such as toilets and food options. Many malls organize walking groups and allow mall walkers in well before the shops are open.

THE GREAT OUTDOORS

If you walk in rural areas, the landscapes can include everything from farmland and forests to hilltops and coastline, and you will be surrounded by the wonderful sights and sounds of the natural world. You may find, too, that spotting birds and other wildlife along the way can pleasantly distract you from the effort you are putting in.

Be prepared, however, as the rough terrain of bridle paths and dirt tracks up hills and across fields may give you a much harder workout than the same distance in a town. There may be less traffic and pollution out of town, but beware of country lanes, because motorists do tend to drive faster there, and the roads can be narrow and without any pavement or verge.

STEPPING IN THE RIGHT DIRECTION

☑ Vary the length of your routes. Even advanced walkers will want shorter routes for when they have less time, or for interval training.

☑ Include surroundings that will suit different moods, from the tranquillity of a park to the bustle of a busy street.

☑ Decide whether you want your walk to start from your front door, or whether you are willing to take transport out to a new area and walk from there.

☑ If walking at night, check that the area is safe, with good pavements and street lighting. Even during the day, avoid known trouble spots.

☑ Avoid busy times on any routes that have heavy traffic and pollution.

☑ Establish the exact locations along your route where you will find toilet and water facilities.

☑ If your walk goes through a public park, check the opening times.

3

Mastering your technique

Now you have your shoes, walking kit, and a safe, well-planned route ready, it's time to work on your technique. In this section, you'll find a step-by-step guide to walking with optimal form. It begins with establishing proper posture, then moves on to mastering the correct arm and leg movements for an efficient walking technique.

Posture

The use of technology in the workplace has led many of us to become more sedentary than ever before, our bodies hunched over desks, reinforcing the very muscles that create poor posture. The best antidote to this is an activity such as walking, where developing good posture is an essential part of the technique.

FUNCTIONAL POSTURE

Your posture is the natural way you hold yourself. Every person's body is slightly different, but without question, better posture can improve your overall health. Without constant and proper use of our core muscles, they become lazy and stop working efficiently. Then, when we do try to stand tall and have good posture, it can feel awkward and uncomfortable because the muscles are being asked to do something they are not used to. Try drawing your navel into your spine and notice how your spine realigns. Doing this regularly will improve your posture and strengthen your abdominal muscles. When your body is aligned it allows your muscles to be used as intended, which will give you more energy, increase lung capacity, and reduce ailments such as back pain. You will also look slimmer and have a more defined shape.

The head-neck-back relationship is key to good posture. If your head juts forwards, your spine will follow suit, straining the muscles in the neck, shoulders, and upper back.

When people start walking regularly they complain of lower back pain and blame it on the exercise when in fact it is caused by poor posture. Correcting posture as early as possible is vital – as we age, bad posture can cause all sorts of problems, from headaches to arthritis.

> **POSTURE TIP**
>
> A good friend gave me this simple tip to correct posture. Attach an elastic band around something you look at often during the day. Each time you see it, spend 30 seconds squeezing your shoulder blades together. Persevere with this and it will become second nature, strengthening your upper back muscles and in turn helping improve your posture.

"Everybody's posture is slightly different, but without question, better posture can improve your overall health."

POSTURE CHECK

Notice how your muscles feel as you bring your body into neutral position.

Incorrect posture The head is thrust forwards, chin jutting out, straining the muscles in the neck and shoulders. The shoulders are slouched and the chest is collapsed. The abdominals are pushed out, arching the spine and throwing the pelvis back.

Correct posture Make sure your weight is evenly distributed, the toes spread to form a stable base. Imagine a straight line from the heel through the back of the knee (not locked). The hips are tilted forwards and the bottom is tucked under. The chest is raised, the shoulders down and relaxed, the neck softly extended. The chin is parallel to the floor and the crown points to the ceiling. The spine is in neutral, which means it is allowed to retain its natural curves.

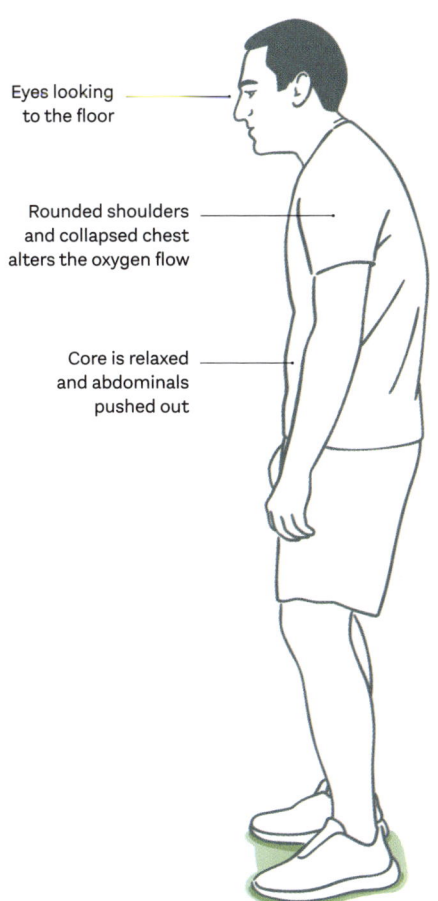

Eyes looking to the floor

Rounded shoulders and collapsed chest alters the oxygen flow

Core is relaxed and abdominals pushed out

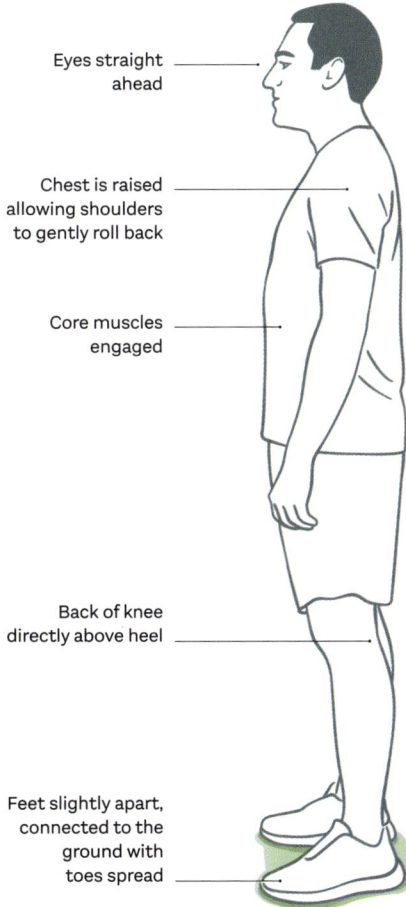

Eyes straight ahead

Chest is raised allowing shoulders to gently roll back

Core muscles engaged

Back of knee directly above heel

Feet slightly apart, connected to the ground with toes spread

MASTERING YOUR TECHNIQUE

Legs

No matter what level you are aiming for, mastering your walking technique will help you to reap the many benefits. Not only will good form improve your posture, strengthen your muscles, and prevent injury, it will allow you to walk faster for longer.

A few minor adjustments to the way you walk will allow you to make the most out of your every step. The action of walking requires the pelvis and hip area to move freely so that the legs can stride out, followed by a pronounced rolling heel-to-toe motion as you move forwards. Work on achieving a strong heel strike and a dynamic push off.

1. Extend one leg immediately while raising the foot slightly in preparation to strike with the heel, as in Step 1. As you practise allow your arms to swing naturally in opposition to your feet (see pp64–65).

2. Taking a normal stride length, with a strong upwards lift on the ankle place your heel squarely on the ground in front of you. This will give a full range of movement as you roll your front foot through to the mid-stance position

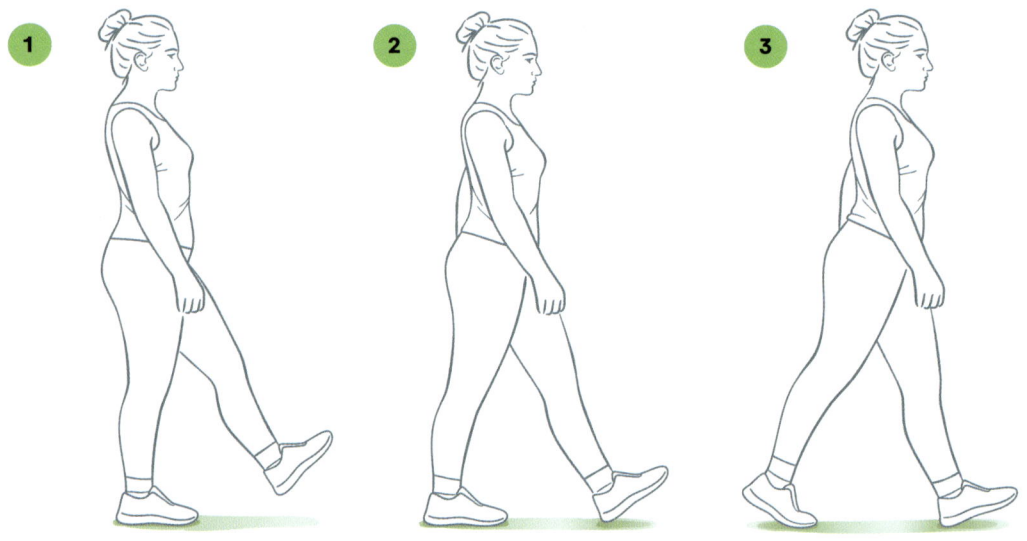

as shown in Step 3. Meanwhile, your back foot is firmly anchored on the ground for stability.

3. As you begin to roll forward onto the front foot, aim to balance your weight evenly between the heel of your front foot and the ball of your back foot, reaching what's called the mid-stance position. Look straight ahead, keeping your chin parallel to the ground. Remember to keep your shoulders relaxed.

4. Transfer your weight onto the front foot, with a straight leg – this is now your anchor. Keep the weight on your left heel for as long as possible before rolling the length of the foot. Begin to lift your heel and rise onto the ball of the back foot ready for your toes to push off; this is the power and energy of every step. It is a challenging move, so begin by exaggerating the push, and feel your back leg extend from your pelvis down to your toes. You may lean forwards slightly at this point.

5. With your front foot as anchor, keeping your foot close to the ground, begin to neatly step the back foot through to the front. Avoid big movements, especially if you want to develop walking fast, as they waste energy and time.

6. Immediately extend your front or right leg, to just above the ground in preparation to strike with the heel as in Step 1. As you practise, allow your arms to swing naturally in opposition to your feet. You will see that it is your arms that give you the momentum to move forward more than your feet!

Walking a line
With each step, imagine that you are walking down an imaginary line. Your feet should be placed almost directly in front of each other, rather than a wide stance. This helps to strengthen your balance, and increase your walking speed.

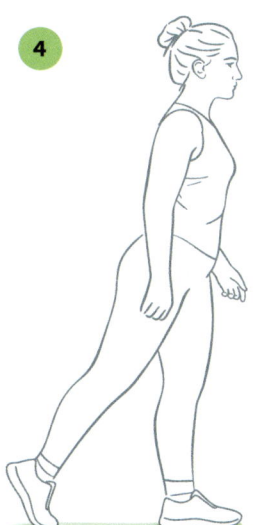
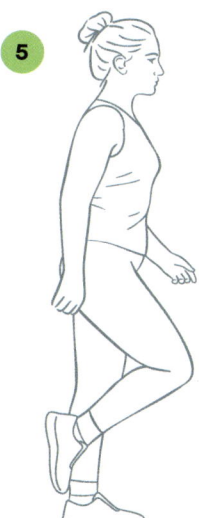
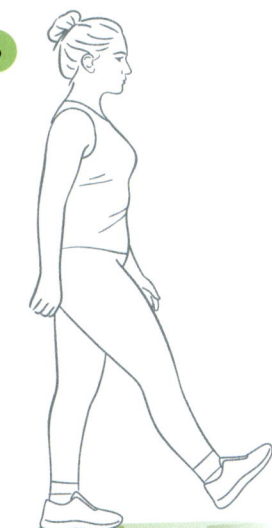

It's all in the arms!

If you have ever tried to walk with your arms fixed to your sides, you will quickly discover you are moving more like a penguin. Your arms offer balance for your legs, and power to your walking, so whether you want to walk in parks for pleasure, or pick up the pace for a marathon, it's all in the arms – the feet can only follow!

1. It is worth experimenting with your arm movements when walking before you leave the house. Stand tall, holding a good starting posture with arms relaxed by your side. Notice what happens with your arms if you walk very slowly, if you walk at a normal pace, and then imagine you are walking fast to catch a bus. Repeat the sequence by keeping your arms by your side. As you begin to refine how you walk, pay careful attention to the natural rhythm of your arm movement in opposition to your steps.

2. If speed is not your aim, then the next step is for you. Start with your arms hanging freely by your sides. Begin walking, with a positive action, allowing your arms to swing back and forth from the shoulder in opposition to your feet. Even if it all feels exaggerated to begin with, using your arms will strengthen all-round mobility and balance. If your fingers start to become swollen, lift them to the Step 3 position and maintain it.

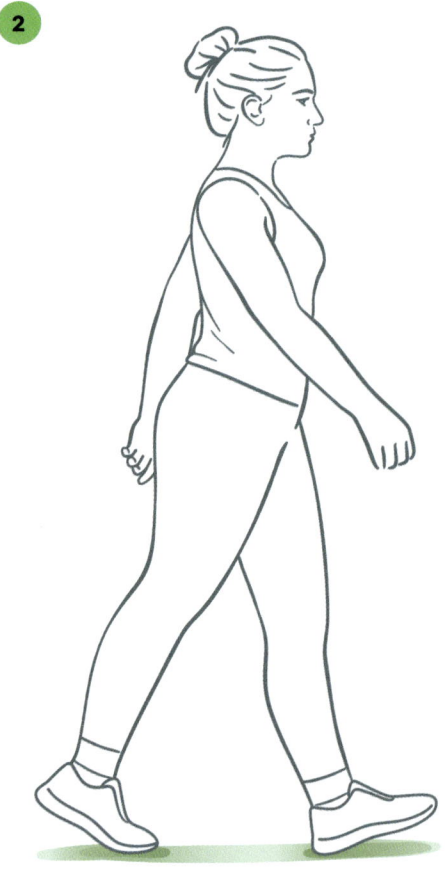

3. This is the neutral starting position for anyone wanting to increase their speed. Your elbows are bent at a 90-degree angle and sit lightly on your waistline. Your hands should be relaxed and gently cupped. From Step 2, get used to walking with your arms in this position, even if you are not actually at the stage of pumping them – that will come. Your elbows remain at right angles, with the pendulum movement coming from the shoulders.

WEIGHTS AND WALKING

I advise against people using wearable weights on wrists or ankles as they can cause muscle imbalance, as well as putting strain on joints and tendons. For an occasional arm workout, try carrying two 500ml (18oz) bottles of water. Alternating between the two and sipping frequently, by the end of your walk the bottles will be empty.

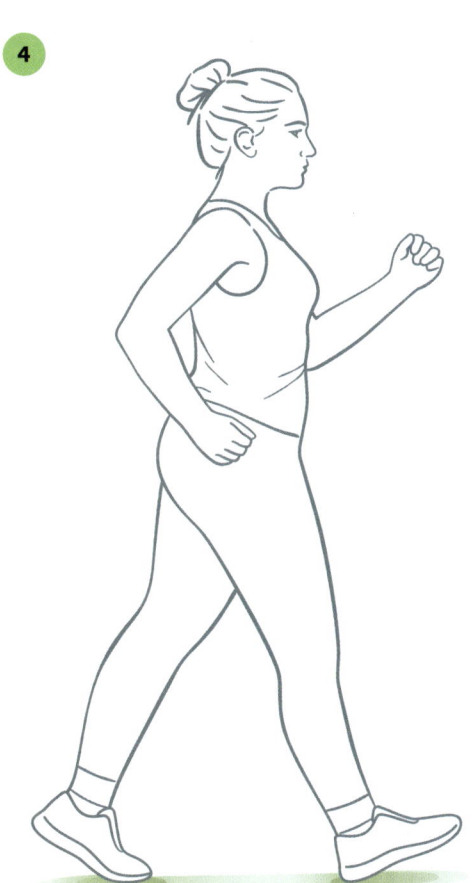

4. You will reach a stage when you begin pumping your arms to move faster. The optimum position is having both arms square to the body and elbows bent at 90 degrees. Practise moving with purpose by pushing your left arm forward as though you are punching the air, your hand reaching no higher than shoulder height. Simultaneously bring your right arm back with force as though you were elbowing someone behind you, keeping your hand just brushing your waist.

Putting it all together

Putting all this technique together, for something that you do every day without thinking, can suddenly feel quite awkward. Considering your posture, the height of your arm movements, engaging your core, keeping your hips square, your eye line ahead, and the actions of your legs and feet, all takes practice to become effortless, but is more than worth it!

1. Begin by setting a good posture, keeping your chin parallel to the ground and eyes looking ahead. Stand with either loose arms by your side, or in the neutral position with elbows bent at a 90-degree angle, depending on the pace you intend to walk. Hands should be soft and lightly cupped.

2. Stride forward on your left leg, with the ankle well flexed. Ensure the back foot is firmly anchored. Start to move the right arm forwards, and the left arm back, in opposition to the feet. As the left heel strikes the ground, begin to transfer your weight from the back foot onto the front foot.

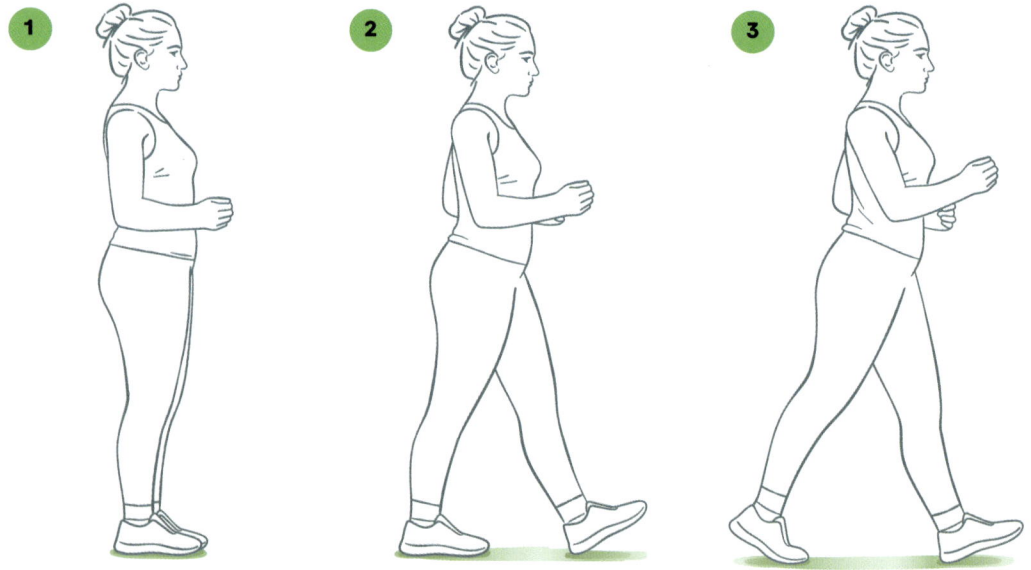

3. At the mid-stance position, your weight is evenly distributed between the ball of the right foot and the heel of the left foot. Continue to move your arms into the optimum position. Make sure you are looking ahead.

4. Transferring your full weight onto your front foot, feel a strong extension in your back leg as your foot lifts onto the ball, the toes ready to give you the power of a good push off, your body leaning forward slightly. At the same time work your arms to propel you forwards, the right arm punching forwards, and the left arm elbowing backwards. Watch that your front hand does not rise above shoulder height, and that the back hand doesn't dip below the waist.

5. With your back foot begin the step through to the front, keeping it close to the ground as you transfer. At the same time, start to move your right arm towards the back and your left arm forwards, again in opposition to the leading foot.

6. Extend the right foot forwards, the toes raised and ready to strike; remember to keep your feet pointing forwards as if walking an imaginary line. Swing the arms through the neutral position and into the next cycle.

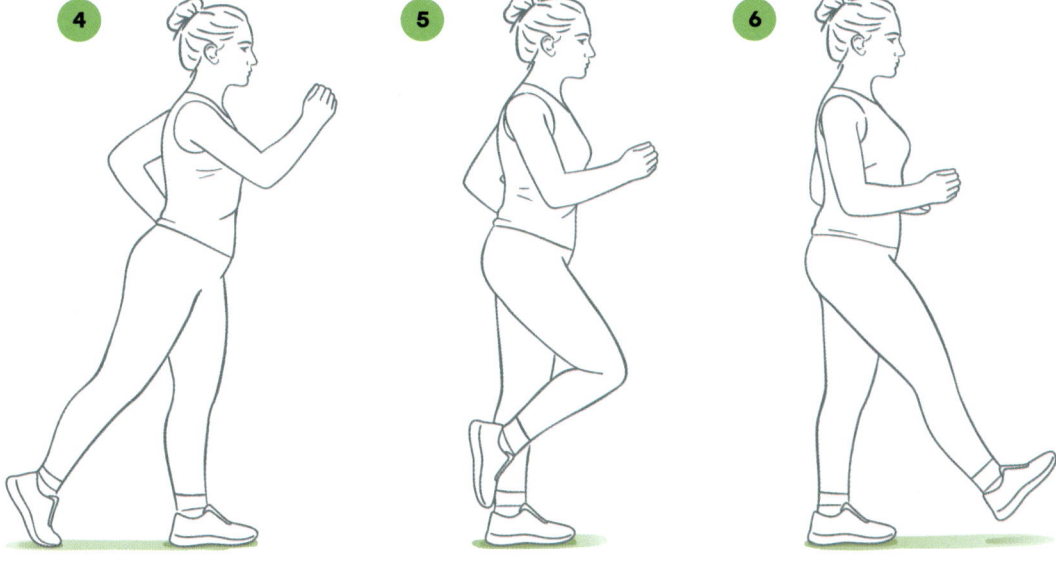

MASTERING YOUR TECHNIQUE

Common mistakes

We are not always conscious of how we walk, until we start to focus in on the detail. Even then, it can be difficult to make adjustments without watching yourself in a mirror or shop window, or asking a friend to give you pointers. Working on posture is always a good start.

Wide and open

A common fault, where arms are held out to the sides, and the foot gait is wide. Men can have a tendency to walk in this way, especially if the lateral muscles are overdeveloped, making it awkward to bring the arms closer. Those with a wide gait can also tend to angle their toes outwards, causing their feet to roll out to the side. Check your shoes support your gait, and actively work on how you are using your feet.

Juggling arms

While the elbows are at the correct angle, the arm going back swings out to the side, as the arm going forwards follows it and crosses the body. Keep your arms at equal widths apart as they pass each other, and keep elbows tucked into your waist. Neither arm should cross the centre line of your body.

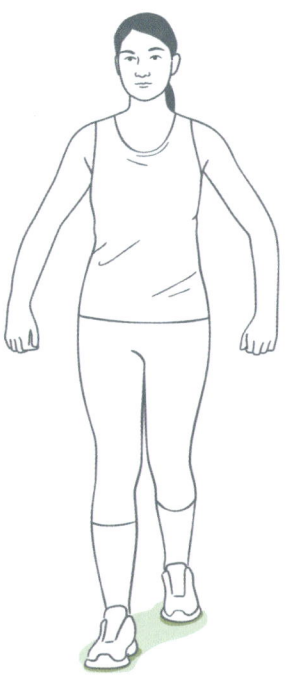
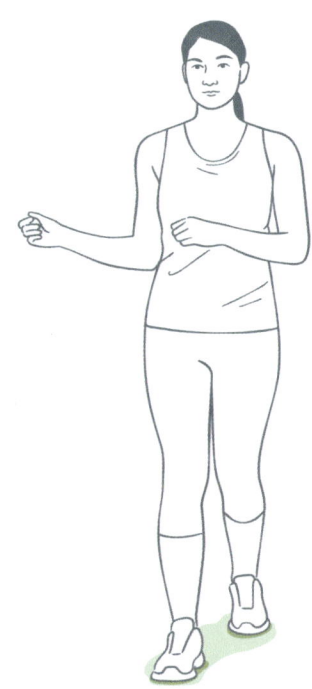

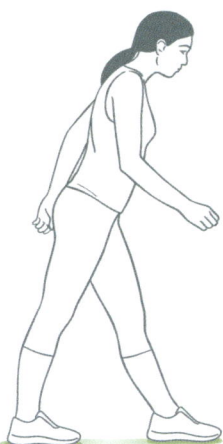 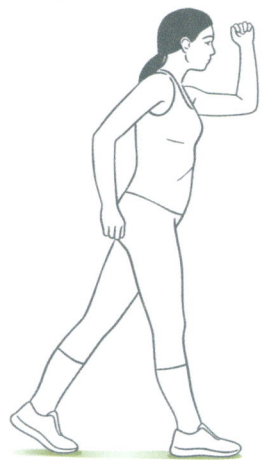

Leaning forwards

This really common fault can stem from overall poor posture, poor technique, or even the habit of constantly looking at your phone. Leaning forwards forces your head to tilt down, which can lead to injuries such as muscle damage and pain in the neck and shoulders. It can also cause lower back pain, which can often be remedied just by correcting your posture. Taking larger than normal strides often accompanies leaning forward, perhaps with the assumption that a longer stride will get you to your destination faster. It actually has the opposite effect; a smaller stride increases the speed. Work on regular posture checks and arm movements, and the feet will follow.

Arms too high or too low

If the leading arm goes too high, the back arm will drop below the waistline. At the same time, your feet may be following in a wider gait. The aim is to be compact, save energy, and allow your arms to give you maximum power. Work on controlling the range of both arms, and check the stride is normal length.

QUICK GUIDE TO GOOD TECHNIQUE

☑ Maintain good posture, engage your core, and avoid leaning forwards.

☑ Ensure a strong upward lift on the ankle of the leading foot as it moves to the heel strike.

☑ Take normal-length strides – don't overstride.

☑ The heel of the leading foot is planted squarely in front of the back foot.

☑ Push off well – this is your power point.

☑ Work your arms from the shoulders, and keep the elbows at right angles at all times.

☑ Keep your movements compact and streamlined.

Staying injury-free

Walking is a low impact exercise, but by strengthening the parts of the body most used – the knees, shins, ankles, and hips – you can help to prevent injuries. If you suffer an injury, only return to intensive walking once your injury has fully recovered. Even then, the damaged area may be susceptible either by weakening or further problems, so take it slowly.

SHIN SPLINTS

Causes and symptoms The calf muscles and the muscles on the front of the shin are probably used more in walking than in any other activity. Walking fast puts pressure on these muscles to work hard. As a result of this, beginners and overambitious experienced walkers can feel a burning, throbbing, or aching sensation, or in milder cases just tenderness, on the front of the shin. Excessive pronation (see p36) can also be a cause.

Usually it is a case of walking too fast or for a longer distance than ability allows. The muscles are being asked to work in a way they are not used to. A common sign of shin splints is that the pain will subside while walking, but will return when you stop.

Treatment and prevention Wrap a bag of frozen peas in a towel and place the ice pack on the shin for around 15 minutes, three times a day, to relieve the muscle ache and reduce any inflammation. To relieve the pain and inflammation you can also use a mentholated ointment such as Tiger Balm, an Epsom salt bath, or an anti-inflammatory. Rest from walking until you feel comfortable again. When you recommence walking, take it gently and slowly build up if you are wanting to walk longer distances or at speed. To prevent this injury from recurring, or from appearing to begin with, it is important to focus on building strength and flexibility in your calf and shin muscles. This can be achieved through regular stretching (see opposite). Start stretching the shins and calves gently every day. Also, look into the fit of your shoes, and check that they are not too big or too tight, causing your toes to grip.

SPRAINS AND STRAINS

Causes and symptoms A sprain is an injury to a ligament that supports a joint and usually occurs as a result of a fall or a twist. This type of injury can range from first degree, which is a stretching of the ligament, to third degree, the complete separation of the ligament from the bone or even a broken bone. Sprains can take weeks or months to heal. A strain is an injury to muscles and tendons. These injuries often result from muscle overuse and can range from a small tear in the muscle to a complete separation of the muscle from the tendon or bone. Both injuries will often result in painful swelling, inflammation, cramping, and weakness. Sometimes you notice the strain at the time it takes place, or you may notice the pain when you have finished your walk.

Quad and ankle stretch

This exercise will help to prevent shin splints and sprains and strains (see opposite), and plantar fasciitis (see p45). Your quads will receive a good stretch and your ankles will be stretched and strengthened as you lift onto your toe. The lift will also strengthen the calves and provide a stretch down the front of the shin.

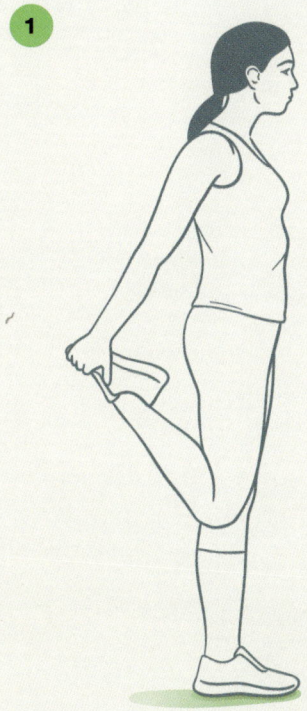

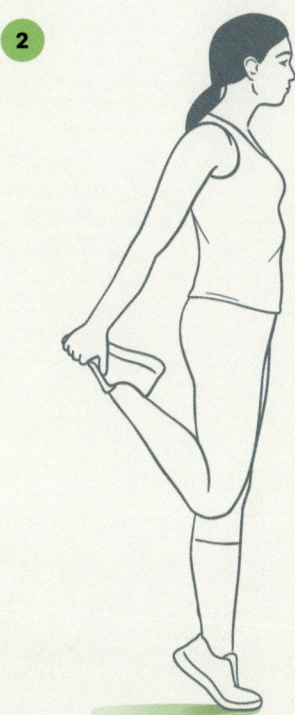

1. Stand with feet a little less than shoulder-width apart, with your arms and hands hanging loosely by your sides. Legs are straight but knees are soft, and not locked. Bring your weight forwards onto the balls of your feet, using your arms to balance you.

2. Using the momentum of your swing and your arms, rock back onto your heels. Ensure knees remain soft. Repeat the rocking motion 5 times forwards and back, rest for 1 minute, then rock forwards and back a further 5 times.

Treatment and prevention Both shin splints and sprains and strains are painful and can be serious, making it difficult to determine the degree of injury and the right course of treatment without professional advice, especially if any anti-inflammatory medication is required. To relieve the immediate pain until advice is available, it is thought that ice packs should be used to reduce swelling, followed by heat therapy promoting the blood flow to reduce inflammation and speed up healing.

Heel-to-toe rock

This exercise helps prevent shin splints and sprains and strains (see p70) by strengthening your shins, calves, and ankles. If you have a weakness in this area, or are a beginner to active walking, you will find doing this for just 5 minutes a day will make a significant difference to your overall stability.

1. Stand with feet a little less than shoulder-width apart, with your arms and hands hanging loosely by your sides, or for support stand in an open door, holding onto each side of the frame. Keeping legs straight without locking the knees, bring your weight forwards onto the balls of your feet, using your arms for balance.

2. Using the momentum of your swing and your arms, rock back onto your heels. Ensure knees remain soft. Repeat the rocking motion 5 times forwards and back, rest for 1 minute, then rock forwards and back a further 5 times.

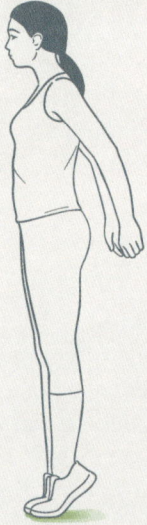
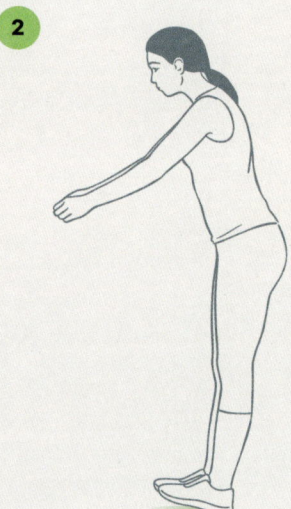

Returning to light controlled movement as soon after the injury as possible is key to recovery. You can also try a mentholated ointment such as Tiger Balm or an Epsom salt bath to relieve the pain and inflammation.

However, once the swelling and pain has subsided, continue with controlled stretching and strengthening (see Chapter 4) on the specific area to keep it mobile and flexible, promoting the joints and muscles to heal.

Wall sit

This isometric low impact exercise promotes joint stability, while building strength and muscular endurance, so is very beneficial for those recovering from an injury or surgery. It is important to breathe slowly throughout, by inhaling through the nose, and exhaling through the mouth.

1 Stand with your head, shoulders, and lower back all flat against a wall. Keep your feet shoulder–width apart, about 61cm (2ft) from the wall.

2 Slowly slide your back down the wall, bending your knees until they reach a 90-degree angle. Thighs should be parallel to the floor, with knees above the ankles. If recovering from injury, work to a depth where the hips are higher than your knees, progressing the movement to lower as you heal.

3 Keeping the core engaged and back pressed against the wall, hold the position for 30–60 seconds or as long as you can hold the form.

4 Slowly straighten your legs, sliding back up the wall, by pushing your mid foot area into the ground. Return to standing.

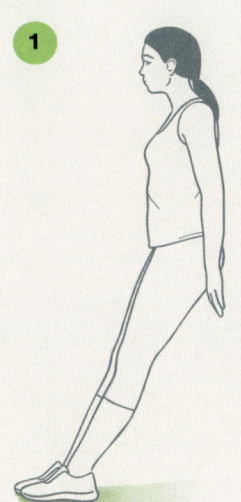

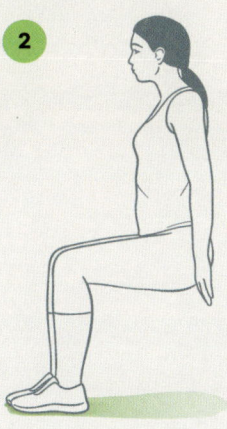

MASTERING YOUR TECHNIQUE

4

Stretch and strengthen

You may be excited with all the walking options ahead of you, but it's important to remember to stretch before and after each walk. Combining walking with stretching and strengthening exercises will enhance your walking ability and make you aware of how your body works, focusing on the importance of core stability.

Why stretch and strengthen?

Our muscular system allows us to perform a range of movements efficiently and without causing stress to the body. Daily stretching before any activity increases blood flow to the muscles, giving greater flexibility and potential to build strength. Stretching after activity reduces risk of injury, eliminates lactic acid, and helps the body relax.

The muscles responsible for movement are known as skeletal, or voluntary muscles and they can act in two ways: they can contract and shorten or they can relax and lengthen. Most skeletal muscles work in pairs. The muscles are attached to bones, so when one muscle group contracts, another muscle group lengthens, pulling the bones together or apart and creating movement. Muscle groups are either mobilizing – creating motion – or stabilizing – holding and supporting while other limbs are moving. This is why it is so important to stretch opposite muscle groups, such as calves and shins, and hamstrings and quadriceps.

FLEXIBILITY AND STRETCHING

Being flexible means that you have good mobility in your muscles and joints. Many factors will have an impact on your flexibility, including your level of activity and whether you work in a sedentary job.

Muscles and joints also become less flexible with age. The way to improve your flexibility, and relieve tension, is through stretching exercises. Before and especially after an activity, stretching is vital to elongate muscles that have contracted through use. Regular stretching, even for just 10 minutes a day, is a good habit to get into, whether or not you have been exercising.

To get the maximum out of your walking, you need flexibility, particularly in the muscle groups you use most: your hamstrings, calves, shins, abdominal corset, and those in your upper back and shoulders.

HOW OFTEN SHOULD I STRETCH?

Try to stretch at some point every day, but always before walking or any kind of activity (see warm up and cool down sequences on p94). For developing strength, follow the sequence of movements on pp80–83 two to three times a week. There is also a specific stretch and strengthening programme you can follow on p95.

CORE STRENGTH

The core muscles in the back and abdomen (see below) help us to stand up and function correctly. In particular, the abdominal muscles, which wrap around the torso and connect the ribcage to the pelvic girdle, keep the core of the body stable and maintain posture. When these muscles are contracted, they act like a corset, keeping the back and front of our bodies in alignment. If these muscles are not used regularly, as in a sedentary lifestyle, they become weak, which leads to poor posture and even shoulder and back problems. By investing in keeping good flexibility and strength, we are not only helping ourselves to stay fit but helping to ensure a long and active life.

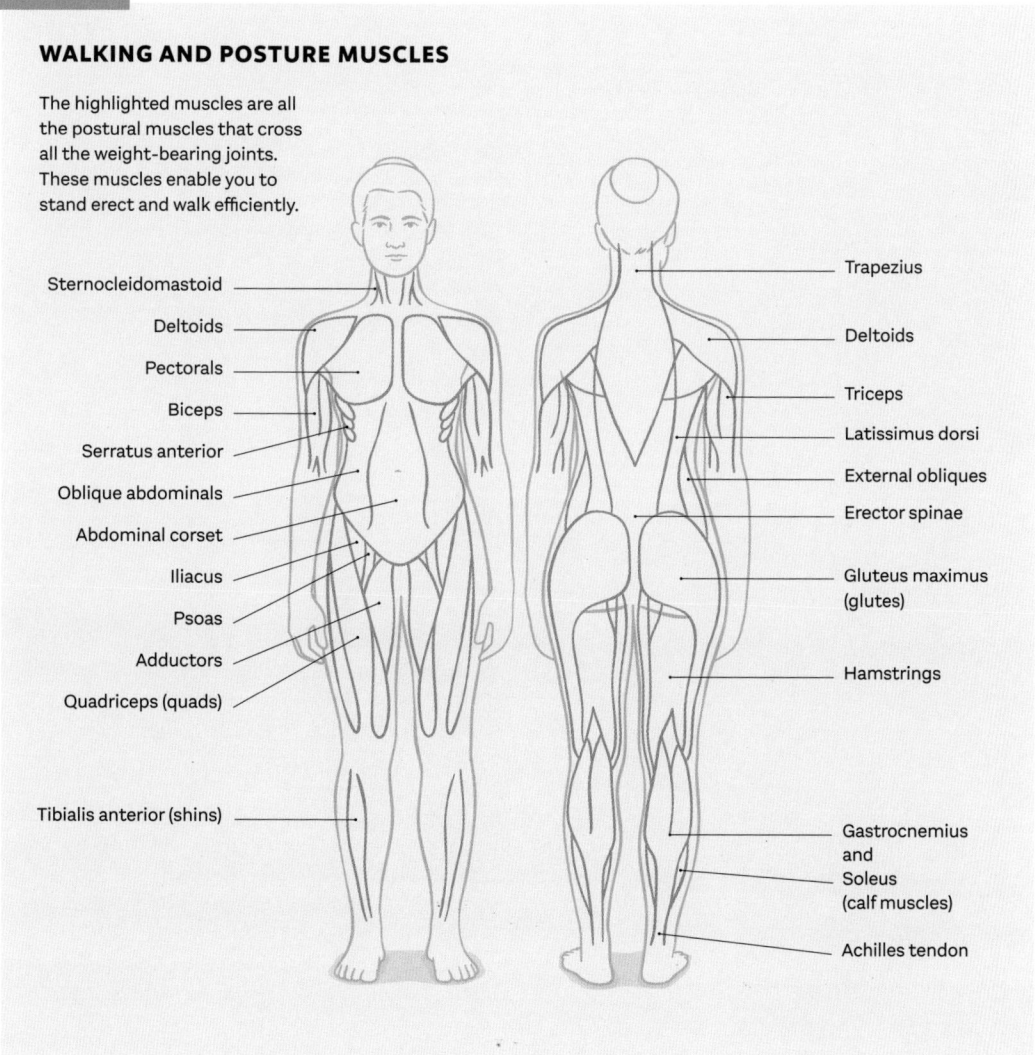

WALKING AND POSTURE MUSCLES

The highlighted muscles are all the postural muscles that cross all the weight-bearing joints. These muscles enable you to stand erect and walk efficiently.

- Sternocleidomastoid
- Deltoids
- Pectorals
- Biceps
- Serratus anterior
- Oblique abdominals
- Abdominal corset
- Iliacus
- Psoas
- Adductors
- Quadriceps (quads)
- Tibialis anterior (shins)
- Trapezius
- Deltoids
- Triceps
- Latissimus dorsi
- External obliques
- Erector spinae
- Gluteus maximus (glutes)
- Hamstrings
- Gastrocnemius and Soleus (calf muscles)
- Achilles tendon

STRETCH AND STRENGTHEN

Stretches for beginners

It's important to start with gentle stretches – you don't want to strain any muscles before you've even left the house! Begin with these two simple stretches, derived from Pilates exercises, to strengthen abdominals and legs.

Double leg stretch

The double leg stretch, a Pilates exercise, is a beginner's stretch and is ideal for strengthening the lower abdominal muscles and challenging your coordination. If you have any problems with your lower back, straighten your legs up to the ceiling in Step 2 instead of holding them at 45 degrees.

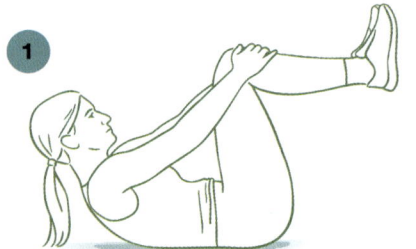

1. Begin by lying flat on the mat, without arching your spine, knees bent with feet on the floor and arms out to your sides, palms facing upwards. Hug both knees towards your chest, keeping elbows wide, and placing your hands on your shins. Keeping your neck long, use your core muscles to lift your head and shoulders off the mat.

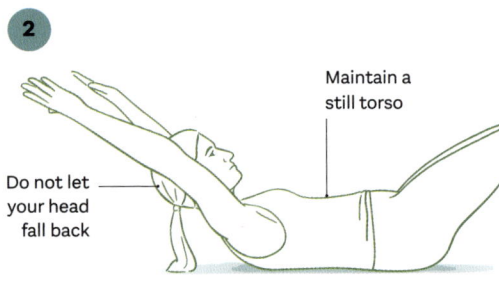

Maintain a still torso

Keep legs straight

Do not let your head fall back

2. Inhale, then stretch out your arms and legs to reach in opposite directions, concentrating on pulling your navel towards your spine. With your toes pointed, hold the position while squeezing your inner thighs.

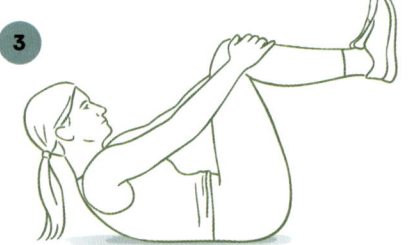

3. Exhale as you bring your legs back in towards your chest and circle your arms to the side and back to holding your shins. Repeat the sequence 5–10 times, keeping the movements flowing and ensuring your lower back is anchored to the floor throughout. If you have back or neck injuries, proceed with caution.

Single straight leg stretch

This Pilates exercise can be completed on its own or following the double leg stretch. It is a more advanced move that strengthens your core muscles and elongates and strengthens the muscles at the backs of the legs. Start slowly, and with practice the action should be quick, smooth, and rhythmic.

1. Lie flat on the mat with knees bent and arms out to the side, palms facing upwards. Hug both knees in to your chest, keeping your elbows wide, and placing your hands on your shins. Using your abdominals, curl your head and shoulders off the floor, bringing your chin towards your chest.

2. Taking hold of the left ankle, extend your left leg up to the ceiling, while stretching the other leg out at 45 degrees from the mat, or at a comfortable height. Pulling your navel towards your spine for support, switch to hold the right ankle as you exhale using a smooth, quick scissor action without jarring the spine. Repeat by completing 5–10 times on alternating legs. Adjust the range of motion to suit your ability.

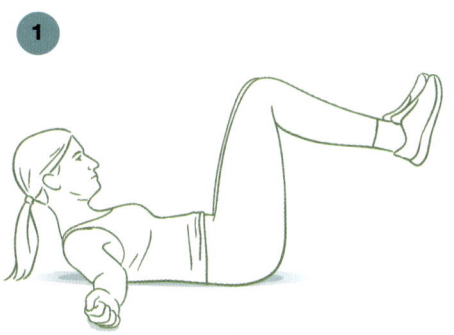

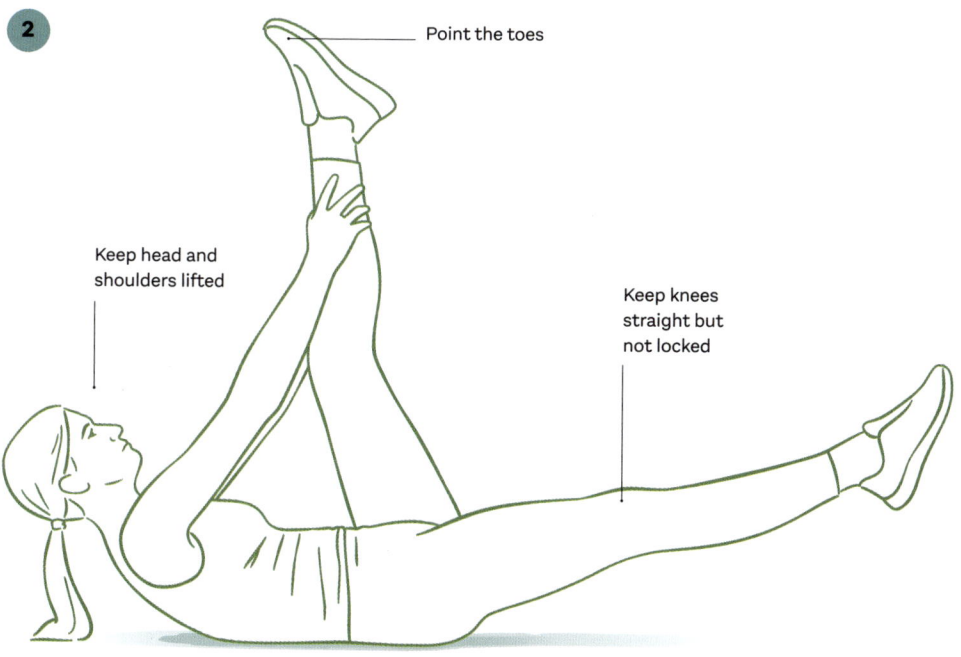

Point the toes

Keep head and shoulders lifted

Keep knees straight but not locked

Developing core strength

Your core is made up of a multitude of muscles including your pelvis, lower back, diaphragm, glutes, hip flexors, and adductors. A strong core is the power behind any activity you do and is fundamental to any carrying, lifting, stretching, and all-round movement in daily life.

A PLANK A DAY!

Easy to perform almost anywhere, the plank is one of the most versatile, multitasking, and all-round body exercises. A plank involves balancing on your toes and forearms or hands, as you hold the rest of your body off the floor. Being weight-bearing, it is good for the bones in the wrists, arms, and shoulders. It also develops muscle endurance, which helps to improve your balance, stability, and posture for sitting, standing, and walking. Plus, it comes with a long list of variations as you progress.

Basic plank

Start in an all-fours position, hands and knees shoulder-width apart on the floor, elbows directly beneath your shoulders so your arms form a 90-degree angle. Extend one leg at a time behind you, with your feet flexed at the toes. Make sure your back is straight and your hips are level. Look directly at the floor in front of you, so that your neck stays in line with your spine. Contract the muscles in the entire area between your ribs and pelvis, reinforcing the straight line from the top of your head all the way to the heels.

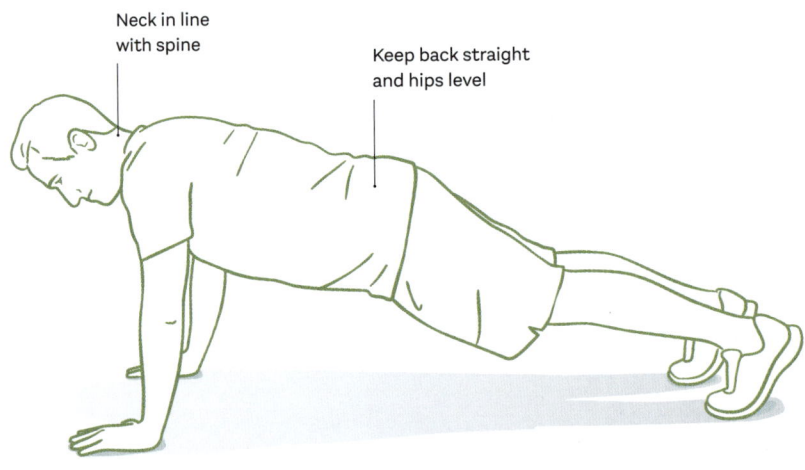

Neck in line with spine

Keep back straight and hips level

Knee plank

For this alternative beginner's option, start with the basic plank, but keep the knees on the floor, placing a cushion under them if required. Support your weight through your forearms or rise up onto your hands, adjusting as required. Cross your ankles and slightly raise your lower legs behind you while pushing your hips up, keeping your spine through to your neck long and straight. Start by holding for 5–10 seconds. As you progress increase to 10–30 seconds. Reaching a maximum of 2 minutes – don't forget to breathe!

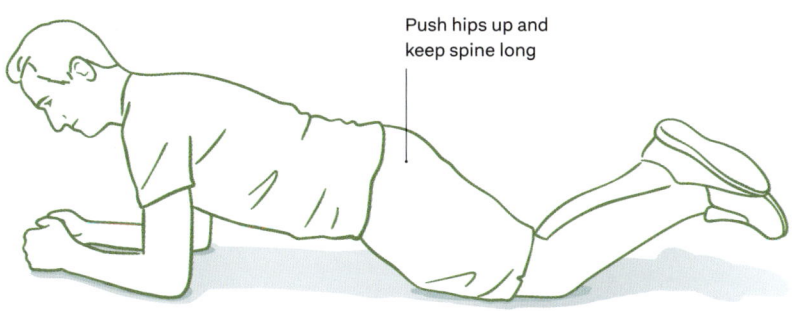

Push hips up and keep spine long

Knee to elbow plank

Begin balancing on hands and toes as for the basic plank, maintaining a tight core and flat back. Bend your left leg, bringing the knee towards your left elbow, pause, and then return to the starting point and change to your left leg. Complete one on each side to start with and build it up slowly.

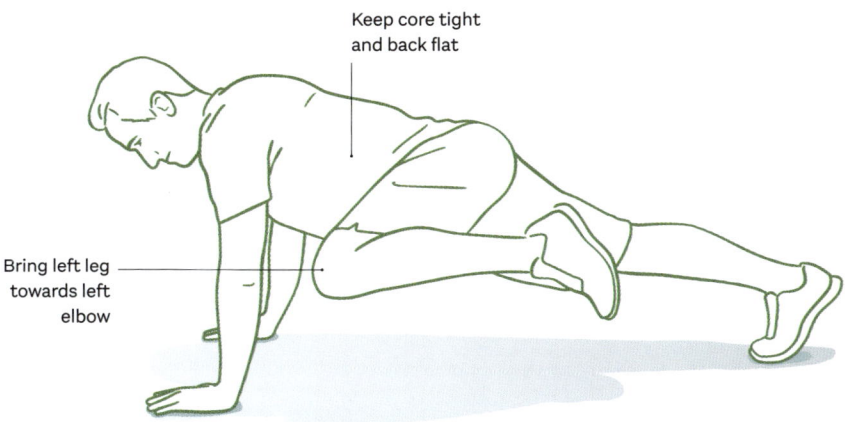

Keep core tight and back flat

Bring left leg towards left elbow

STRETCH AND STRENGTHEN

Knee to nose plank

Begin in the basic plank position (see p80), rising up onto your hands as well as your toes. Arch your back, drop your head, and bring your right knee towards your nose. Return the right leg to the starting position and swap to repeat on the left leg, keeping a smooth steady rhythm.

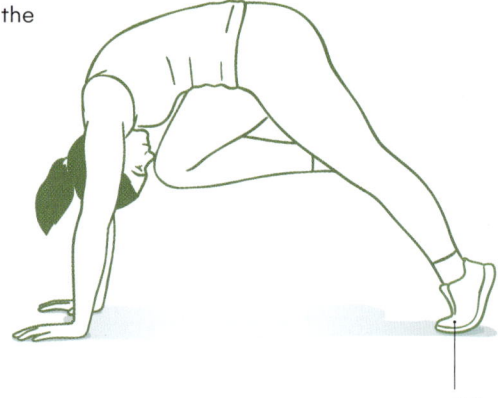

Balance on toes

Bird dog plank

Begin in the basic plank position (see p80), balancing on your hands and toes, facing downwards, and back straight. Raise your left leg off the floor straight behind you, at the same time as raising your right arm off the floor straight in front of you at shoulder height. Repeat on the other side, stretching your right leg behind you and your left arm in front.

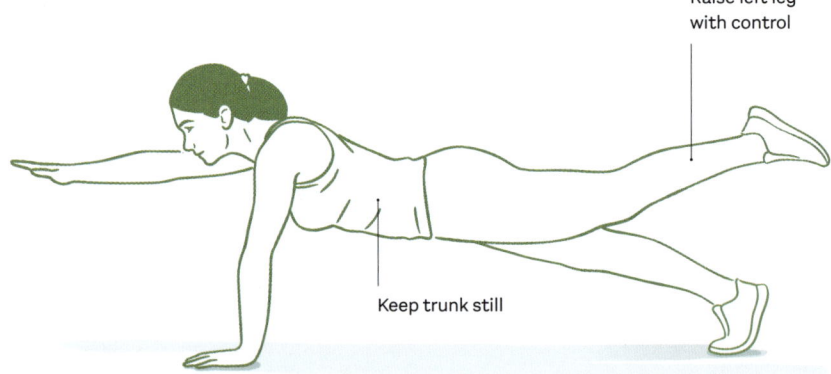

Raise left leg with control

Keep trunk still

Reverse plank

Once you have mastered the basic plank (see p80), you can try the reverse plank, which will build strength along the back of your body.

Begin by sitting on the floor with your legs extended in front of you. Place your palms (with fingers spread wide) on the floor, slightly behind and outside of your hips.

Pushing into your palms, lift your hips and torso while keeping your arms and legs straight and your toes pointed. At the same time, tilt your head back and look towards the ceiling. You should be forming a strong straight line from head to toe.

Hold the position for 30 seconds, or as long as you are able to hold the stance correctly. Then lower yourself back to the starting position.

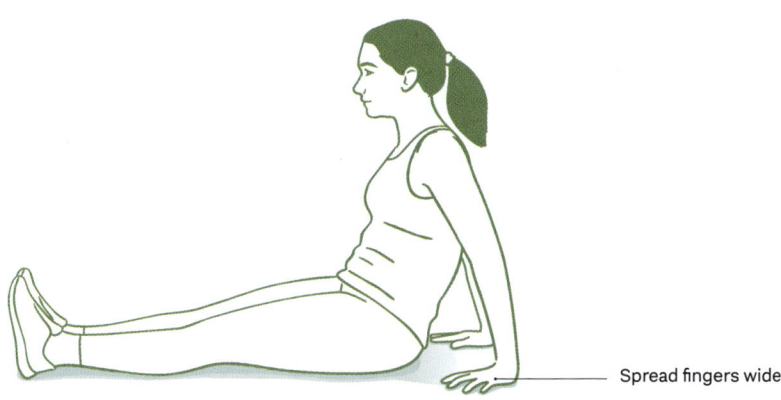

Spread fingers wide

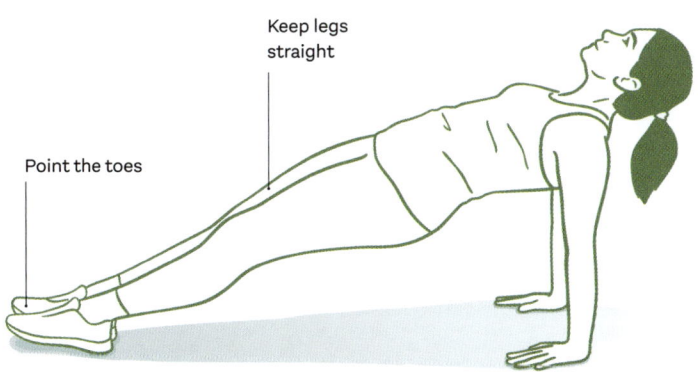

Keep legs straight

Point the toes

Upper body stretches

The upper body, shoulders, arms, chest, and neck can hold a great deal of tension, which can cause stiffness. Stretching restores good mobility and releases stress. These upper body stretches are subtle but effective. They should feel pleasurable, so if they are painful in any way, you are pushing too hard. Be aware of having good posture before beginning each stretch.

Neck stretch

Stand tall with your feet slightly apart and knees soft. Move your arms behind your back, with your right hand lightly clasping your left wrist. Keep the shoulders straight and gently ease the left arm towards your right arm. You should feel the stretch at the front of the left shoulder. Hold for 10 seconds and repeat for the other arm.

Alternative
Tilt your head to the right as you ease the left arm towards the right. You should feel a stretch all the way down the left side of your torso. Hold for 10 seconds, then repeat the entire sequence on the other side.

Triceps stretch

Stand tall with knees soft and legs hip-width apart. Raise your left arm above your head and bend it so that your hand is pointing down your spine. Place your right hand on your left elbow and gently ease your left elbow backwards to get a good stretch in the back of your arm. Hold the stretch for 10 seconds and then repeat for the other arm.

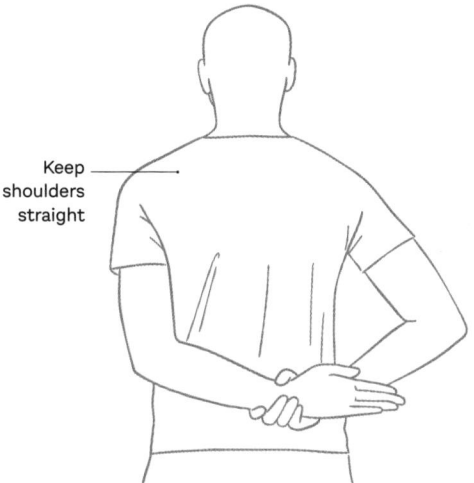

Keep shoulders straight

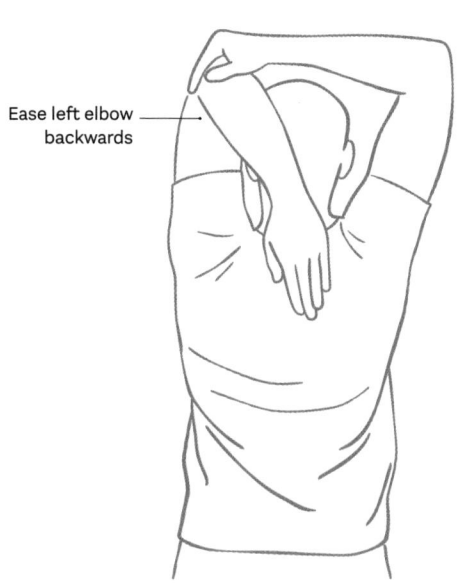

Ease left elbow backwards

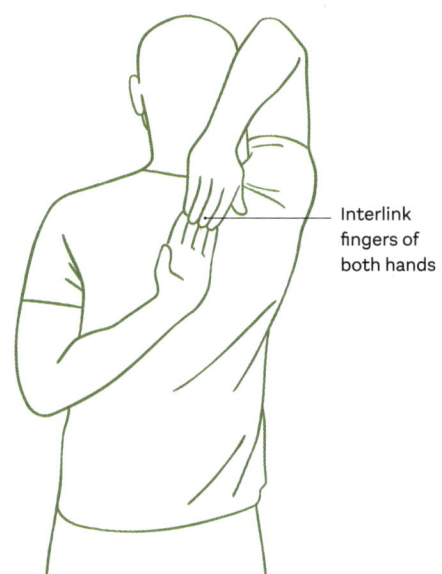

Interlink fingers of both hands

Shoulder stretch

Stand tall with knees soft, and reach up with both arms. Feel a stretch lifting from the pelvis all the way up to your fingertips. Keep your right arm raised and bend it so that your hand is pointing down your spine, palm facing in. Drop your left arm, bend the elbow and interlink the fingers of both hands. Check that your back is in neutral and not arched. Feel the stretch through both shoulders while you hold for approximately 20 seconds, then repeat with opposite arms.

Beginner's alternative
If you are unable to reach far enough to interlink your fingers, hold a belt or small towel to bridge the gap; gradually work at bringing your hands together.

Upper back stretch

This stretch releases tension in the upper back, shoulders, and neck. Kneel on the floor with knees approximately hip-width apart. Lean forwards to place your hands in front of your knees, palms facing downwards. Walk your hands forwards away from you until your arms are outstretched. Feel the stretch through your spine from your pelvis and deep in your shoulders. Hold for 15 seconds and then return to a sitting position.

Alternative
Poor flexibility and tightness in your shoulders and upper back can prevent you from enjoying the full stretch. If this is the case, fold your arms on top of each other and rest your head on your arms. Open your shoulder blades and feel a gentle stretch in your upper back.

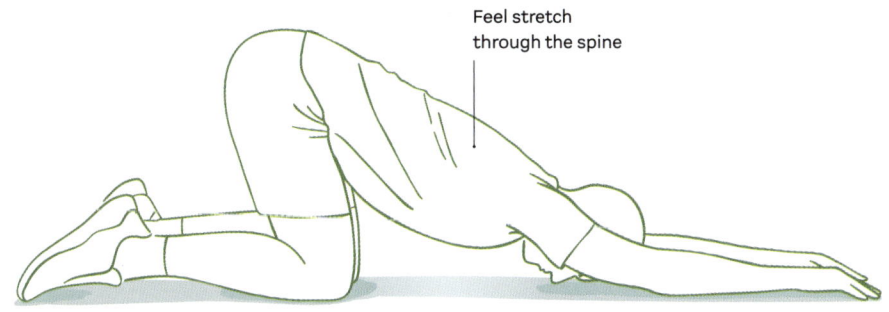

Feel stretch through the spine

Lower body stretches

The muscles and joints in the legs, pelvis, and lower back are going to work hard while walking, so they need particular attention. It is important to build strength in vulnerable areas, such as knees and ankles, to reduce the risk of injury. Focus on the actual muscles you are stretching, and complete the routine as regularly as you can.

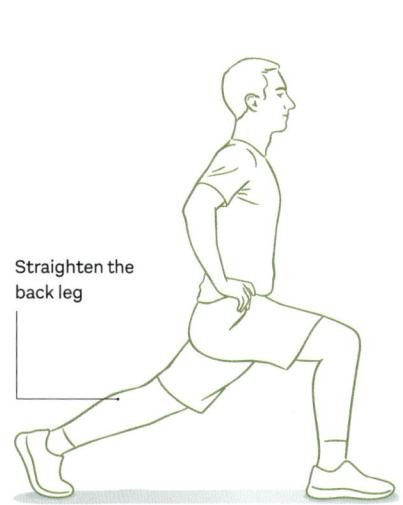

Straighten the back leg

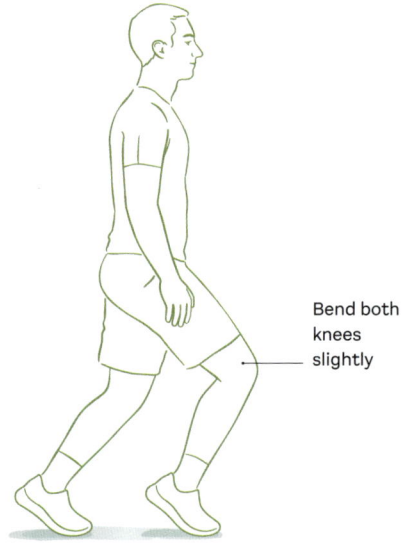

Bend both knees slightly

Standing hip flexor lunge
Stand tall with your feet hip-width apart, then take a step back with your left leg. Place your hands on your hips for support. Lunge slowly forwards onto your right leg, keeping the knee at 90 degrees and above the heel, while straightening the back leg. Keep hips square and ease them forwards by tightening your buttocks, then stretch in the front of the hip. Hold for 10 seconds then switch sides.

Hip flexor stretch
Begin with a staggered stance, one foot in front of another. Lift your chest, bend the knees slightly, and raising your heels while keeping hips square. Tilt the hips gently forward without arching your back. Pull back to the starting position and change sides.

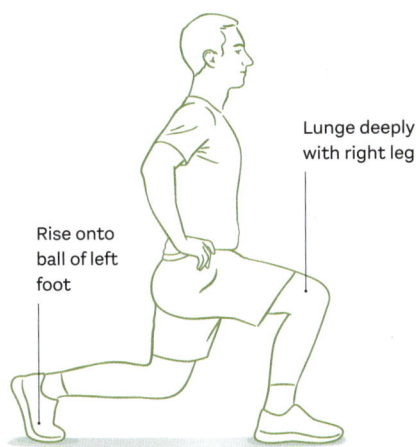
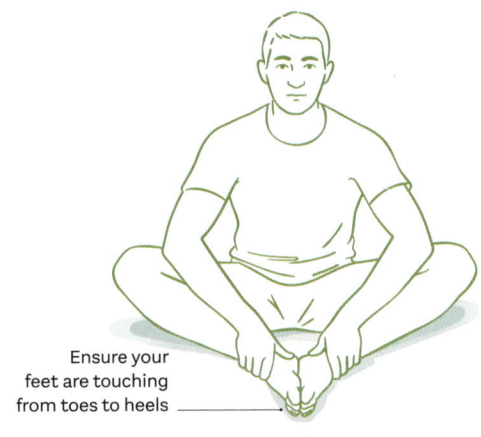

Achilles tendon stretch
Stand tall with your feet hip-width apart, then take a step back with your left leg. Lean forwards on the right leg into a deep lunge as though you were going in to the Hip Flexor Stretch. Then rise up onto the ball of your left foot to create a good stretch for the Achilles tendon. Hold this for 10 seconds and repeat on the other leg. This stretch works well when completed following on from standing Hip Flexor Lunge.

Ankle stretch
This yoga stretch is ideal for walkers as it increases flexibility and strengthens the ankles, knees, and hips. Sit up straight on the floor, raise your chest, and place the soles of your feet together, placing hands on ankles and elbows onto your inner thighs. Gently push your elbows out to feel the stretch through the inner thigh.

Hamstring and calf stretch
Stand tall, with your feet together. Step your left leg forwards a normal stride length. Stand with your right foot flat on the floor, toes pointing ahead and left foot flexed. Bend your right knee and place both your hands at the top of your right thigh to support your weight. Lean forwards slightly onto your right foot and sit back into the position. Feel the stretch in your hamstring and calf. To intensify the stretch, sit further back. Hold for 10 seconds and then repeat on the other side.

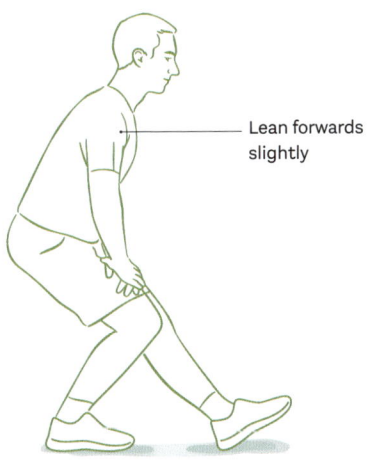

Full body stretches

The side rolls rotate the spine and stretch your obliques (the waist muscles). To advance the side rolls, grip a tennis ball between the knees. This will keep your pelvis straight and stretch your obliques more intensely. The back stretch gives the spine a powerful stretch and opens the chest.

Side rolls

Lie flat on the mat with your knees bent at a 90-degree angle, knees close together. Stretch your arms out to the sides, palms facing downwards (A). Inhale deeply, and as you exhale, slowly turn your head to the right. At the same time, slowly and in a controlled movement, roll both legs to the left (B). Hold the stretch for about 15 seconds, return to the start position, and then repeat on the other side.

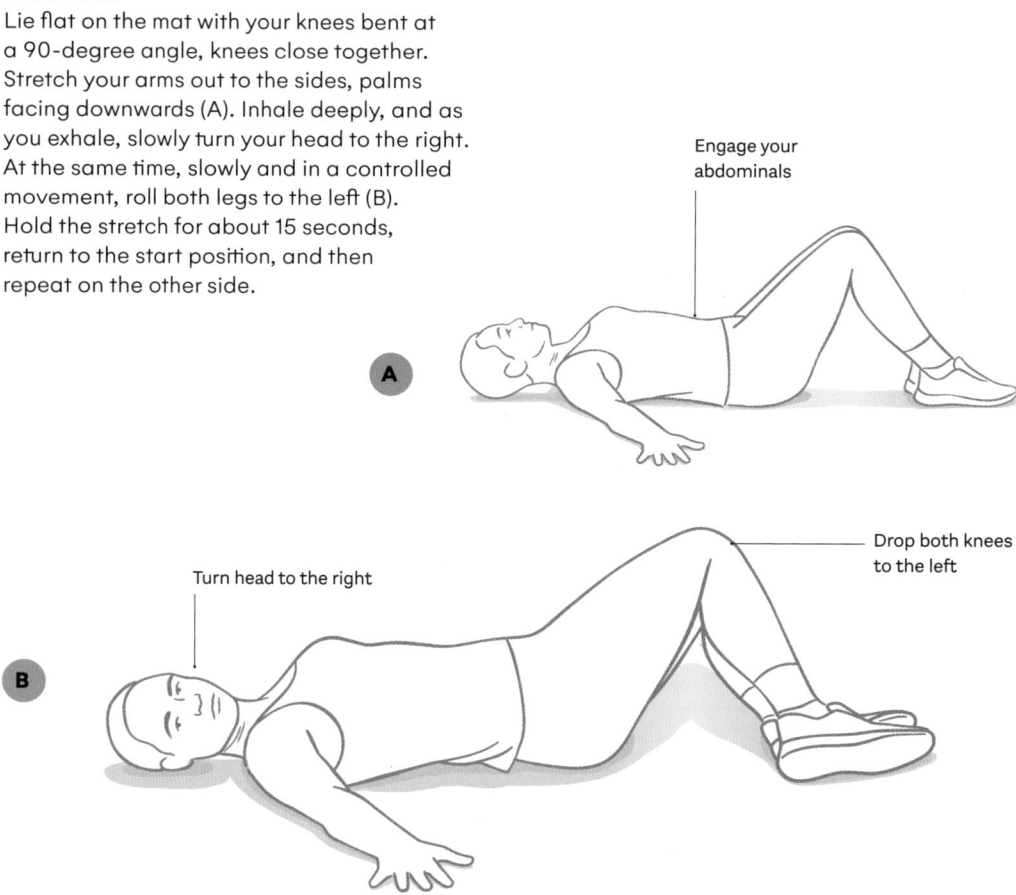

Back stretch

Lie on your front and place your hands directly under your shoulders, with elbows bent and arms close to your sides. Push up from your hands, but keep your elbows bent at around 90 degrees. Hold for 10 seconds, feeling the stretch right down your back. Avoid this exercise if you have any sensitivity or problems in your back.

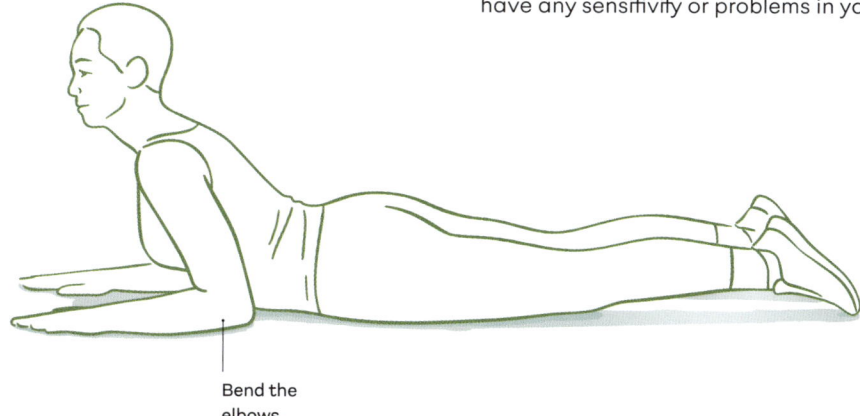

Bend the elbows

Advanced stretch

From the lying position, push up with your hands as before. Continue to raise your chest and shoulders, lifting from your hips and midsection, until your arms are straight but your elbows are not locked. Your shoulders should be relaxed, shoulder blades dropped down. Hold for 10 seconds, then return to the start position.

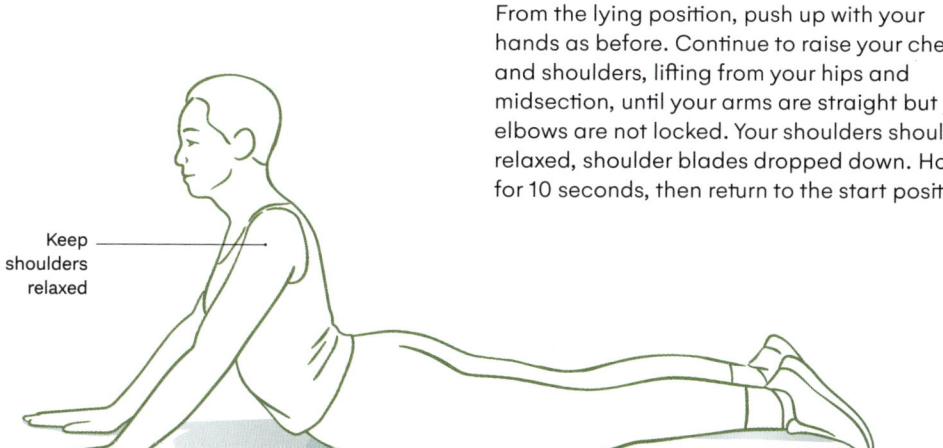

Keep shoulders relaxed

Before and after walking

Warming up and cooling down are essential to prevent aching and injuries to muscles during and after exercise. A short routine will aid flexibility and increase the blood flow into muscles. Once the muscles are soft and warm, stretching will lengthen them and train them to become more pliable. Make these exercises a key part of any walking programme.

WARMING UP

Warming up prepares the body to be active. As you gently exert yourself, your temperature rises and your blood begins to move more rapidly towards the muscles that are being used, increasing their flexibility. Tight muscles are underused muscles and prone to injury.

If you are quite fit, begin your warm up by walking at an easy pace for 5 minutes. If you are planning a long, demanding walk or if you are unfit you will need a minimum of 10 minutes. Keeping your eyes focused on the path ahead, start to loosen your shoulders and the upper body as you walk, rolling your shoulders a few times. Swing your arms in circular movements and an exaggerated pendulum motion. Your lower body will become warm through the movement of walking. Focus on your body and become sensitive to how it is feeling at that moment. After 5–10 minutes find a suitable spot to stop and follow the warm-up sequence (see p94). Taking deep breaths, relax into holding each position for 10–15 seconds. There should be no pain or pressure, just the sensation of your muscles lengthening. When you have finished, continue walking, increasing your pace gradually over the next 5–10 minutes. If you feel tight during the course of the walk, slow down and stretch again.

MIND AND BODY

Warming up not only prepares your body for movement, it also puts you in the right frame of mind for exercising. After a hard day's work, for example, the last thing you feel like doing is pounding the streets. A few minutes of gentle walking and stretching has a miraculous way of changing your mind. Conversely, cooling down allows you time to calm and centre yourself before launching back into life.

COOLING DOWN

The longer and more intense your workout, the longer your cool down will need to be. It is not a good idea to abruptly stop walking as this can cause dizziness. Five to ten minutes before the end of your walk, begin cooling down. Slow your pace, and once again roll your shoulders and swing your arms. When you stop, follow the cool-down sequence (see p94). This time you can make the stretches deeper and more intense, holding the positions for 15–30 seconds.

With each inhale and exhale focus your breath to the muscles your are stretching, allowing the breath to release any tension. Do not bounce as this can cause strains. Take care not to overstretch because this can cause a weakness in your joints. It should feel comfortable, not painful. If you know that you have weak areas, work specifically on those places. End your session by relaxing in the corpse pose (p93) – not always possible but a treat when you can.

The tree

This yoga position is good for developing your balance while also calming and refreshing the mind. Although it is an unusual choice, I find it is excellent for cooling down and becoming centred. To help you balance, place one hand on a wall for support.

1. This exercise should be performed in bare feet. Stand tall with your feet just slightly apart, your toes spread and your weight evenly balanced between both feet. Transfer your weight onto your left foot and clasp your right ankle. Place the heel of your right foot as high as possible on the inside of your left thigh with your toes pointing down.

2. Focus on an object in front of you, and stretch your arms out to the sides at shoulder height to help your balance. Keep the right knee pointing out to the side and your hips straight. If you feel comfortable, raise your arms in a wide, open gesture towards the ceiling. Keep strong and rooted, yet flexible and relaxed. Hold this position for about 10 seconds and then repeat on the other side.

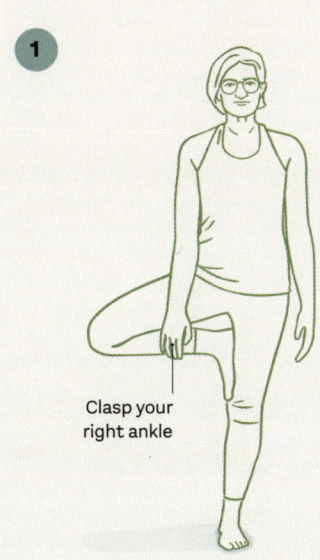

Clasp your right ankle

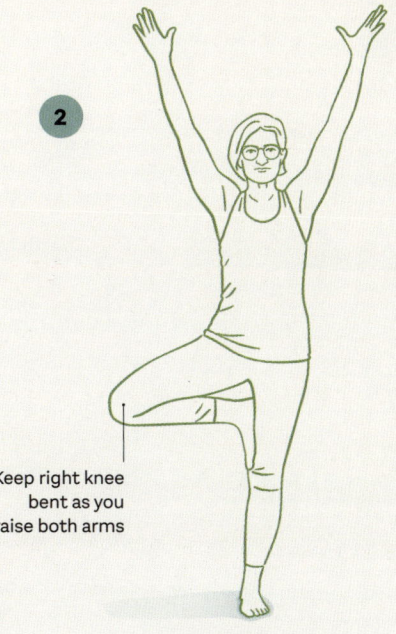

Keep right knee bent as you raise both arms

Back stretch roll down

A supple and flexible back is important for your health and fundamental to any movements that you make. Our backs can become tight, not only from lack of use but also from stress, so spend just a few minutes each day repeating these exercises, which will benefit your walk and day-to-day health.

1. Stand tall with your feet slightly apart, a stride's length from a wall. Inhale, and raising your arms above your head, reach high to lengthen your spine.

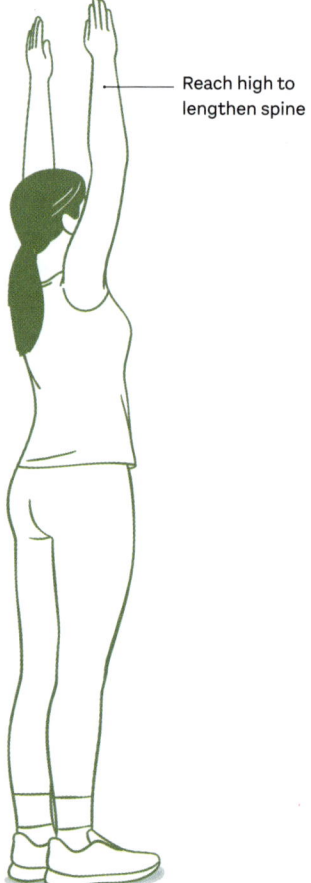

Reach high to lengthen spine

2. As you exhale, slowly roll down from the pelvis. Reaching out with your hands, place them on the wall so that your back is parallel to the floor. Feel the stretch through your back.

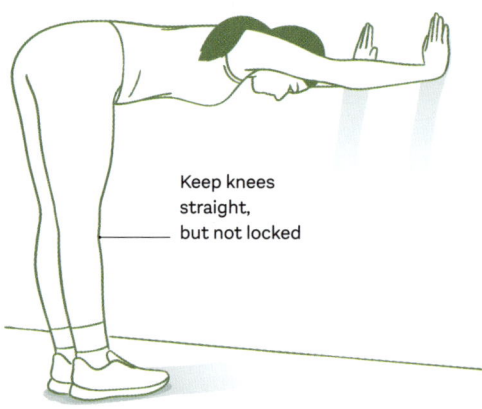

Keep knees straight, but not locked

3. Exhale deeply and allow your body to drop towards the floor. Feel the stretch through each vertebra of your spine and the backs of your legs. Hold for a few seconds, then slowly curl up along the length of your spine to return to a standing position.

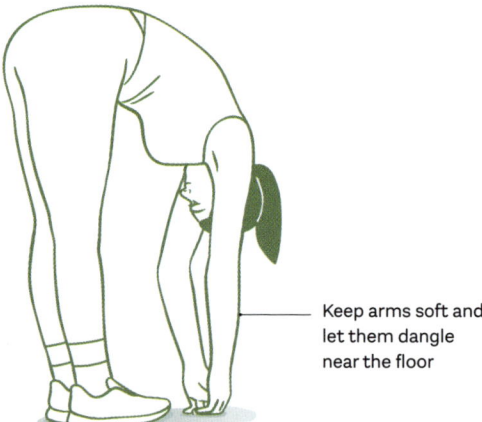

Keep arms soft and let them dangle near the floor

Calf stretch

Stand tall and position yourself facing a wall or doorway. Press the ball of your left foot against the wall with your ankle at a steep angle. Keep hips square, facing front and directly above the heel. Inhale deeply and as you exhale ease into the stretch in your calf. Hold for a few seconds, then repeat on the other leg. Alternate legs, stretching for a total of 5 times on each leg.

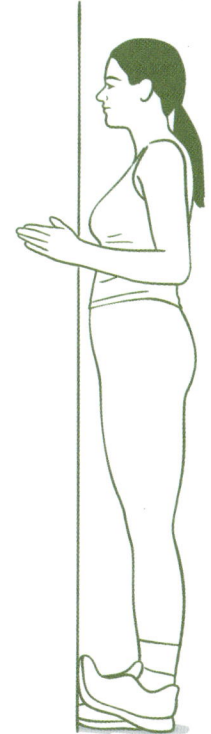

Corpse pose

This yoga pose can release stress from the spine, leaving the body calm and centred. Lie on your back with your legs slightly apart, arms away from your body with palms facing upwards, eyes closed. Allow your body to feel soft and relaxed. Imagine your breath reaching areas of tension. Remain in the pose for up to 10 minutes, then stretch your arms, roll onto your side, and slowly come up into a sitting position.

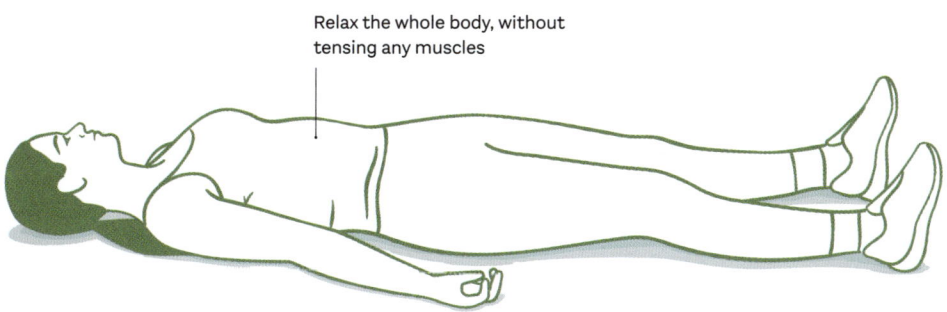

Relax the whole body, without tensing any muscles

Warm up and cool down routine

Warming up before any activity increases the blood flow to your muscles, reducing the risk of injury. Cooling down allows for your blood pressure and heart rate to reduce gradually to pre-activity levels.

Warm-up sequence

Walk at an easy pace for around 5 minutes and then do each of these stretches in the order shown. Hold each position for 10–15 seconds. Distance walkers and those beginning a fitness programme will need to walk for 10 minutes before stretching.

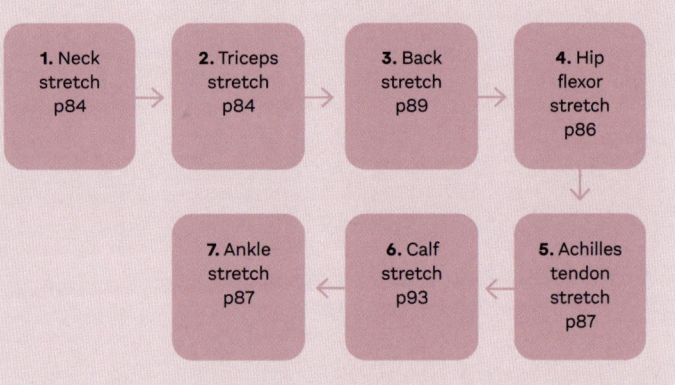

Cool-down sequence

Begin your cool down by slowing your pace 5–10 minutes before the end of your walk, then do each of these stretches in the order shown for a full cool down. To ensure a deeper stretch, you need to hold each position for 15–30 seconds.

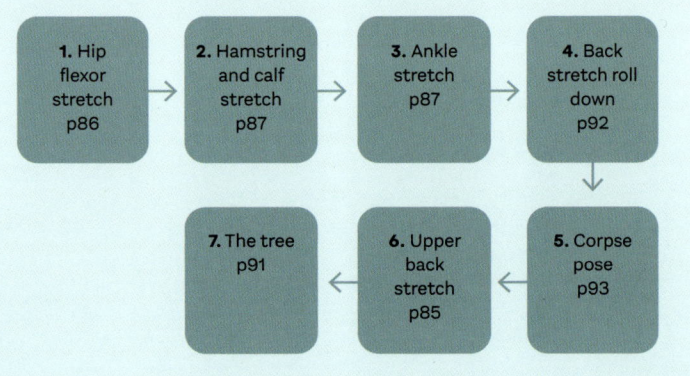

Stretch and strengthen routine

Daily stretching will not only help to retain your flexibility, it will also develop muscle endurance.

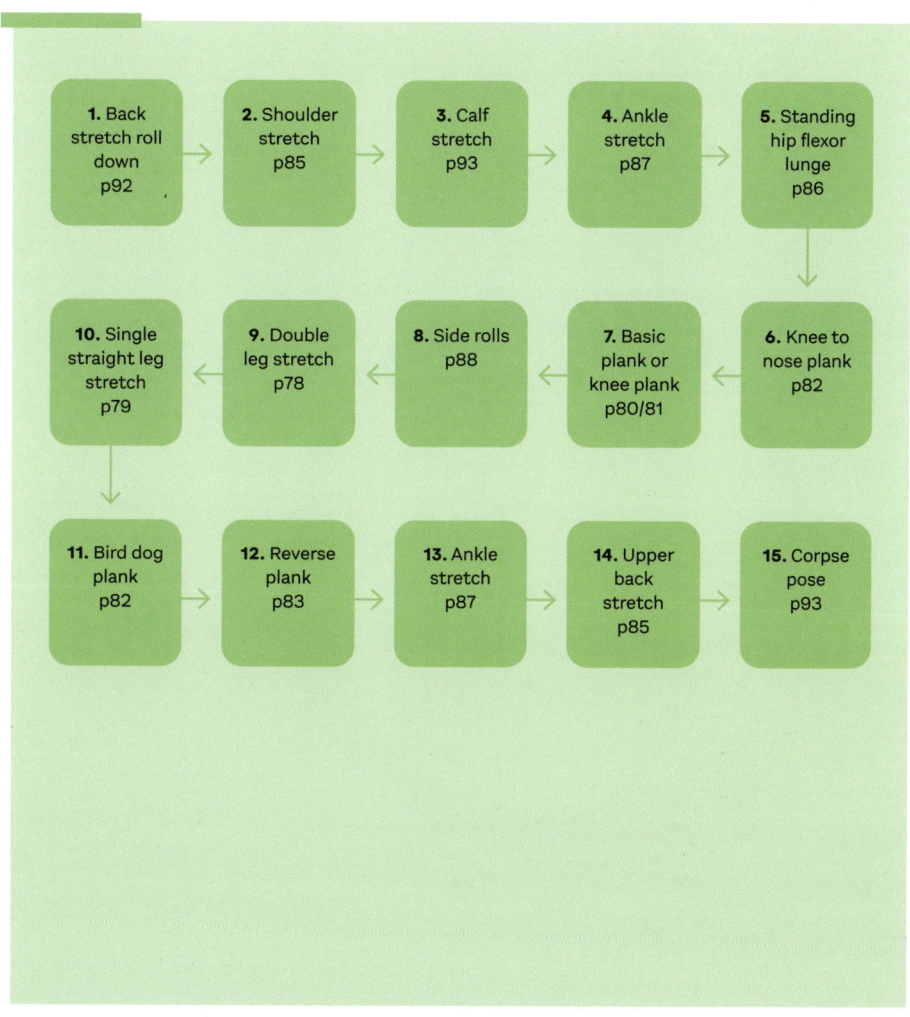

5

Caring for your mind and body

Regular activity brings many benefits, but supporting your physical and mental wellbeing is essential, too. Breathing, body awareness, and positive thinking, as well as foot care, combined with a healthy diet and good hydration, will all help you meet your walking goals.

The power of breath

Without realizing it, many of us take very shallow breaths through the mouth, and use only the top of the lungs. By breathing more fully and deeply, we can gain more energy, vitality, and enthusiasm for life. It will enhance how we walk, and contribute to our emotional wellbeing too.

BREATHING

The act of breathing is so natural that most of us don't give it a second thought. Yet few of us breathe correctly. In general, people use shallow, or chest, breathing and do not use the full capacity of their lungs. Poor posture, too, can restrict the ribcage and prevent the lungs from expanding properly.

Breathing deeply using the diaphragm when you are walking will help you to get the most out of your sessions (see p101 for more on diaphragmatic breathing). But first you need to get in touch with your breath and experience the energy it brings.

Try the breathing exercise opposite, and as you breathe, mentally send oxygen into the body. Feel the sensation of directing air in and out while the spine lengthens. Practise this until you are able to recreate the feeling when you are out walking.

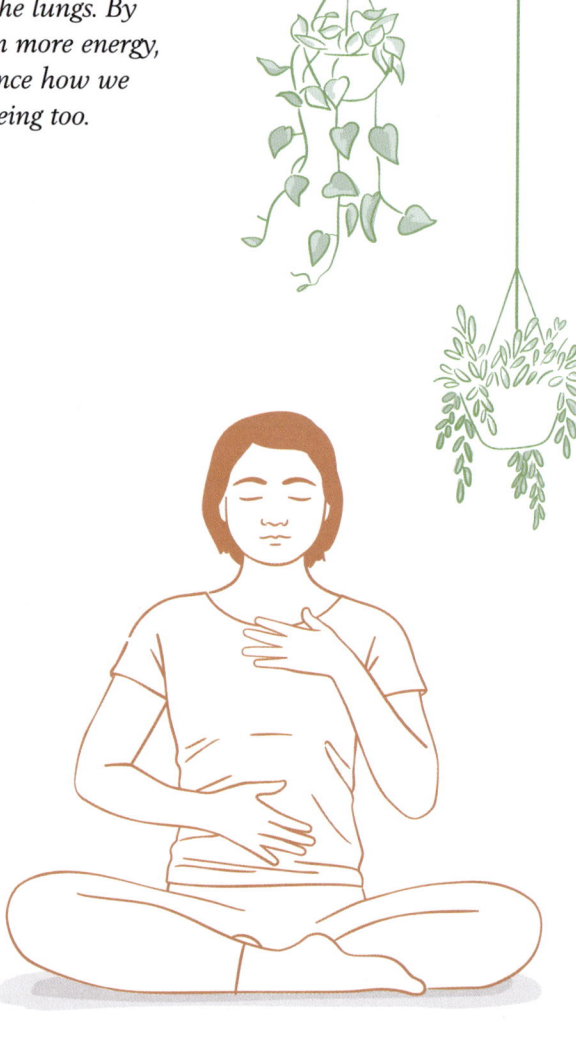

Breath awareness

Lie on your back. Lengthen your neck by bringing the chin slightly towards your chest. Feel your belly button pulling towards the spine. Place one hand on your abdominals just below your navel and the other on your ribcage. Breathe in slowly and rhythmically and be aware of the corset muscles working. Do not allow the abdomen to pop out. Breathe out and feel the sensation of your ribcage moving. Widen the shoulders and feel the shoulder blades moving slightly towards each other. Experience the whole of your upper body broadening rather than moving upwards.

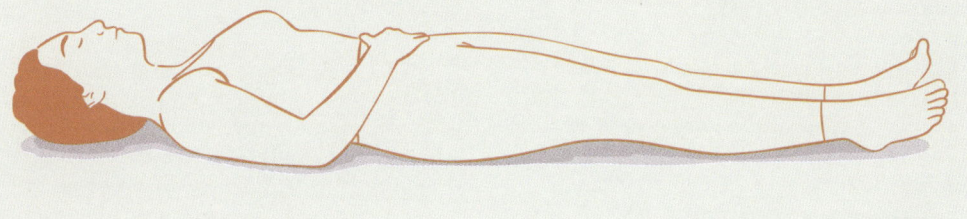

THE MIND-BODY LINK

The act of breathing supports a strong mind-body connection. We know that our state of mind can affect our breathing patterns. When we are frightened or angry, our breath speeds up and becomes irregular. In a totally relaxed state, our breathing becomes slow and rhythmic. In the same way, how we breathe habitually can affect our mood. Shallow breathing through the chest closely resembles the breathing of someone in a state of anxiety, and disrupts the right balance of oxygen and carbon dioxide needed for a relaxed state. Ancient yogis remind us that when the breath is deep and calm, the mind is still, and to achieve this most of us have to work on improving our breathing.

"The act of breathing supports a strong mind-body connection."

THE DEMANDS OF EXERCISE

It can be quite a struggle, for example, when we are exercising and we find ourselves puffing and panting away. The key is to practise proper breathing before working out, and once on the move, to focus on inhaling and exhaling rhythmically so as not to hyperventilate, which deprives the body of oxygen. The body needs more oxygen when you exercise, and you will find that you naturally increase the number of breaths you take per minute, but you should still maintain a rhythmic cycle of breathing. There is no more exhilarating feeling than when your shoulders are back and relaxed, your chest is open, and your breathing is deep and easy – you will feel that you could walk effortlessly for a hundred miles!

Before working out

Rhythmic breathing: This is a conscious and deliberate breathing pattern, with the ultimate goal of synchronizing your breath with your body's natural rhythm. It can offer emotional balance, mental clarity, and improved physical health.

1. Find somewhere comfortable and quiet to sit with your feet placed flat on the floor. Try inhaling in for 4 seconds and exhaling for an equal count.

2. Alternatively, try inhaling for 4 seconds, holding your breath for 7, and exhaling for 8.

Be aware – as with all breathwork, if you have any medical conditions it is always best to seek medical advice before starting.

On the move

Pursed lip breathing: Adjusting the rhythm, and the way you breathe while walking, can, over time, improve your lung capacity, strength, and power. Pursed lip breathing helps you to inhale and exhale more air, and to slow your breathing. As you increase your heart rate, pursed lips reduce stress, making it easier to exhale.

1. Slowly inhale through your nose before the muscle lengthening part of the walking motion – such as extending your leg for the heel strike (see pp62–63).

2. Gently exhale completely through tightly pursed lips during the shortening part of the motion as you bring the back foot forwards.

3. Keep good posture to allow the space in your lungs to fully expand.

4. If you experience a side stitch while walking, try exhaling during the left footfall (not the right).

ABDOMINAL BREATHING

To oxygenate the body fully, we must breathe deeply using the diaphragm (children breathe like this naturally). This is often referred to as diaphragmatic or abdominal breathing. The diaphragm is a muscle situated between the chest and abdomen. When you breathe in, it moves down to make room in the chest for the lungs to fill with oxygen. As you breathe out, the diaphragm moves up, reducing the chest size, and squeezing air out of the lungs. You are breathing correctly when your abdomen swells forwards as you breathe in, and gently falls as you breathe out, and there is little or no movement in the chest area. Remember, breathing out is just as important as breathing in. The more stale air that you can get rid of as you breathe out, the more clean air you can take in.

Diaphragmatic breathing

Diaphragmatic, or belly breathing, helps to strengthen your diaphragm muscle, which contracts to pull air into the lungs. This type of breathing improves the amount of oxygen entering your blood from your lungs with each breath. It can increase your body's ability to exercise as well as form the basis for any relaxation.

1. Lie on your back, knees bent for support, and using a pillow under your head.

2. Place one hand on your upper chest, and the other on your belly just below the ribcage.

3. Inhale slowly through your nose. As the air reaches your lower belly, your hand should rise, while the hand on your chest remains still.

4. As you exhale through pursed lips, tighten your abdominal muscles, letting them fall inwards. The hand on the belly moves to the original position.

5. Practise for 5–10 minutes a few times a day.

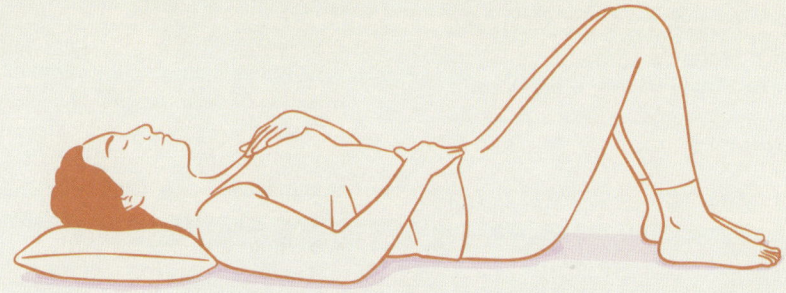

A positive mindset

You can apply the principles of a positive mindset to any area of your life – not just your fitness journey. The mind's power to affect physical health has been much talked about, but is there any proof? Well, psychologists in the USA have found that people who feel positive about ageing live on average 7½ years longer than those who see only its downside.

Clearly, the power of thought can have a big influence on our lives, for better or worse. We all hold a constant inner dialogue, or self-talk, that can switch from positive to negative and back again. It is often easier to follow the negative path, telling ourselves that we are going to fail or that things won't go right. This prevents us from looking forward to events with happy anticipation, and we may even end up bringing about the very thing we fear.

That negative inner voice can not only prevent us from having the optimism to try to achieve our full potential, but it can also affect our health. Research in Canada carried out over 30 years shows that patients who expect to do well after an operation recover more quickly than those with a pessimistic attitude.

CHANGING YOUR INNER VOICE

So how can we change our attitudes to use the beneficial power of the mind? The first step in making the change is to become aware of the nature of our own inner voice.

Psychologists believe that an average person experiences between 20,000 and 60,000 thoughts a day. None of these thoughts are neutral: they are either positive or negative, and they will reinforce themselves day after day.

If you are one of the people who always sees a glass as half empty rather than half full, you need a positive inner voice to describe your life as you would like it to be. A good way to begin changing your mindset is to repeat positive affirmations (see opposite).

You will greatly increase your chances of success if you not only believe 100 per cent that you will achieve your goal, but you have a goal that is realistic and achievable, one that creates a challenge for you, but is not impossible to fulfil.

CHANGING NEGATIVE THOUGHTS

Reframe your thoughts by changing how you view yourself and how you describe yourself to other people. For example, saying "I'm stupid" will in time make this part of your identity. Instead, think in terms of behaviour, which can be changed. You may sometimes do stupid things, but no one is infallibly wise. Forgive yourself for your mistake and think of the successes that can be balanced against it.

It is important to remember that positive thinking will not magic away the negative things in your life, but it will help you to create more positive outcomes.

AFFIRMATIONS

Our minds are fickle; it is not always easy to keep our thoughts on the matter in hand. Practising affirmations is a powerful tool. Using this technique will help you to stay positive, focused, and keep believing in your own abilities. Always affirm the positive things that you desire, and not negative outcomes that you are wanting to prevent, keeping them personal and in the present tense. Make them realistic, so that you can say them with sincerity, and make them in the present tense. Instead of saying, "In six months time I want to feel fitter," say, "Every day in every way I am fitter and stronger." Never have more than two or three affirmations at any time, giving each one time to work on the subconscious.

It is the self-belief and constant repetition of affirmations that produces the results, and there is no better time to do them than when you are out walking. Let them fall in tune with your step, and repeat them again and again, like a mantra (see p129).

VISUALIZATIONS

Like affirmations, practising visualizations is about conditioning your mind by repetition, but this time using images and sensations rather than words. You may find it easier in the beginning to close your eyes so that you are not distracted by the reality around you. The more you practise, the clearer the images will become and the more your subconscious mind will accept them as the truth, banishing any underlying negativity that may be holding you back. For example, if you are planning to take part in a marathon, imagine yourself reaching the finish line, smiling and strong. Feel the breeze on your face as you walk and hear the crowds cheering you on. Think about the clothes you are wearing and how they feel against your skin, and imagine the surge of joy that courses through you when you receive your medal at the end. Try to create a full-colour picture in your mind, including every little detail exactly as you want the experience to be. The more times you return to this powerful image, the more likely it is to become reality.

Be body aware

If we take our bodies for granted, we risk ignoring the warning signals they send out in the form of aches and pains when we have overexercised or suffered an injury. In this book, you will learn how to recognize, treat, and prevent some of the most common walking injuries. By listening to your body and sticking to a few rules, you should stay injury-free.

As you start walking, you will naturally become more aware of your body, and the effect being active has on it, both positive and negative. Pay attention to your body so that you know how it feels when it is functioning normally. You will then find it easier to recognize if something is not right.

RECOGNIZING THE SIGNS

Mild aches and pains are the body's early-warning system. Learn how to read these signs so you can decide whether it is better to take a break that day. It may be that a self-treatment at home is all that is required, but if you are in doubt and the pain becomes severe or chronic, err on the side of caution and seek medical advice.

While low impact, walking can exacerbate old injuries that were possibly not treated properly at the time. Alternatively, you may discover that you have uncovered a muscular or postural imbalance that was also not evident before. In either of these instances, discuss the problem with your doctor.

Keeping a record is a good way of tracking your overall health. Try recording details such as how far you walk, what pace, and how you feel, both mentally and physically. Also noticing any aches, pains, or concerns, will help you to address them before they become serious.

YOUR SUPPORT TEAM

Build a support team that can assist you in keeping your body strong and healthy. My support team includes a chiropractor – always my first port of call – an acupuncturist, a chiropodist, and my doctor. Research these practitioners in advance so that you have someone to turn to if you do have an injury.

Visit health specialists for maintenance sessions, not just when you experience pain. Lower back pain is common in power walkers and is usually due to a poor walking posture by leaning forward from the hips. Checking your technique and visiting your chiropractor can help.

SCANNING YOUR BODY

Using a body-scan meditation teaches you the skill of moving through your body and becoming sensitive to any physical changes.

- Sit comfortably and shake out any tension in your limbs and torso. Take some deep breaths.

- Begin by focusing on the area at the top of your head, then move down over the scalp and forehead, noting any tightness or pressure.

- Check that your eyes are soft and your mouth, tongue, and jaw are relaxed.

- Continue moving down your neck, into your throat, and then into the shoulders, arms, and hands. Again, note any subtle sensations.

- Feel the movement in your ribs and diaphragm with each in and out breath.

- As you focus on your belly and your lower back, notice your posture and any discomfort.

- Focus on your hips, legs, and feet. Feel your feet firmly planted on the ground. Throughout the scan, breathe normally. If you find an area of tension, keep your awareness there until you feel the knots dissolve away. You may like to repeat the head-to-toe check one or more times, each time going deeper into relaxation.

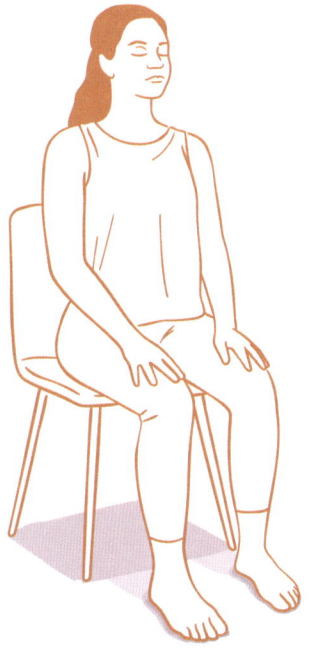

CHECKLIST FOR WALKING WELL

Walking is a low-impact sport, so injuries are few and most are very preventable, provided you listen to your body and follow a few simple rules:

☑ **Footwear** Wear the right shoes and socks that will support your feet and the type of walking that you intend to do (see pp38–49).

☑ **Warm up and cool down** Stretched and activated muscles are much less likely to suffer injuries. Don't forget to bring muscles back to their resting state after exercise (see p94).

☑ **Stretching and strengthening** Make it a habit to stretch every day, allowing your muscles the ability to develop a full range of motion (see Chapter 3). Follow a strengthening programme that suits your ability.

☑ **Change is as good as a rest** Whatever your goal, if you walk fast or a long distance one day, go for a shorter meditational walk the next, or even do something entirely different. Cross training with dancing, swimming, or free weights gives your body a change.

☑ **Consistency** Being impatient or over-ambitious by going too fast, too far, and too soon will lead you to discomfort. Pace yourself, walk within your ability, and feel yourself progress, which is far more motivating!

☑ **Change your terrain** If you usually walk on roads, try taking yourself on a hill walk or on softer ground such as grass. Treadmills are also good for a soft surface but not nearly as exciting.

☑ **Give your feet some attention** Having any foot problems can be enough to spoil your walk or even cancel it. Remove any rough skin, which can cause blisters, and cut toenails with rounded corners so they can't catch on the toe next to it. A great walk begins with caring for your feet (see pp106–109).

How to massage your feet

Massaging your feet is a powerful way to ease tension and relax your whole body. There is no time limit, but a minimum of 5–6 repetitions of each movement is much more relaxing than moving onto the next step too quickly. You will need essential oils, a base oil such as almond oil, and two towels.

1. Make up a massage oil consisting of 3 drops to 10ml (2 tsp) base oil. A combination of lavender, marjoram, and neroli oils makes a very relaxing mix. Prepare your hands by putting a few drops of oil into your palms and massaging your hands together until they feel soft and warm. Hold your foot sandwiched between your hands for a few moments, then stroke your foot with gentle sweeps towards your body, one hand behind the other.

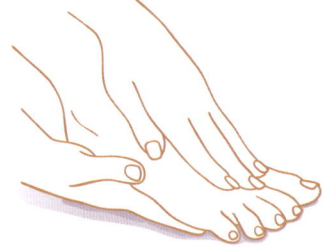

2. Massage each toe using your thumbs. Continue by gliding your thumbs along the top of your foot towards your ankle and then back towards your toes, fanning your thumbs out to the side as you glide.

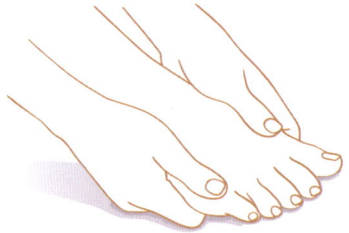

3. Start to loosen your toes by sandwiching them between your palms and rotating them clockwise and then anti-clockwise.

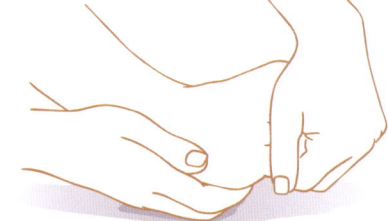

Be aware – always check with a qualified aromatherapist before using any essential oils during pregnancy or if you have a medical condition. Use almond oil on its own if you are unsure.

4. Massage each toe again, this time with your thumb and forefinger, giving them a light squeeze and a roll. Finally, gently pull each toe in turn towards you.

5. Using gliding movements, run your thumbs between the four tendons on the top of your foot, moving towards the ankle.

6. Firmly massage the sole of your foot. Use your thumbs to ease out from the centre to the outer edges. Find a good reflexology book to tell you more about the powerful effect that massaging points on the feet has on the rest of your body.

7. Massage around the ankle and Achilles tendon area, making small firm rotations. This feels instantly relaxing as we hold a great deal of tension in our ankles. Complete the massage by stroking the foot. Wrap it in a warm towel or blanket while you work on the other foot.

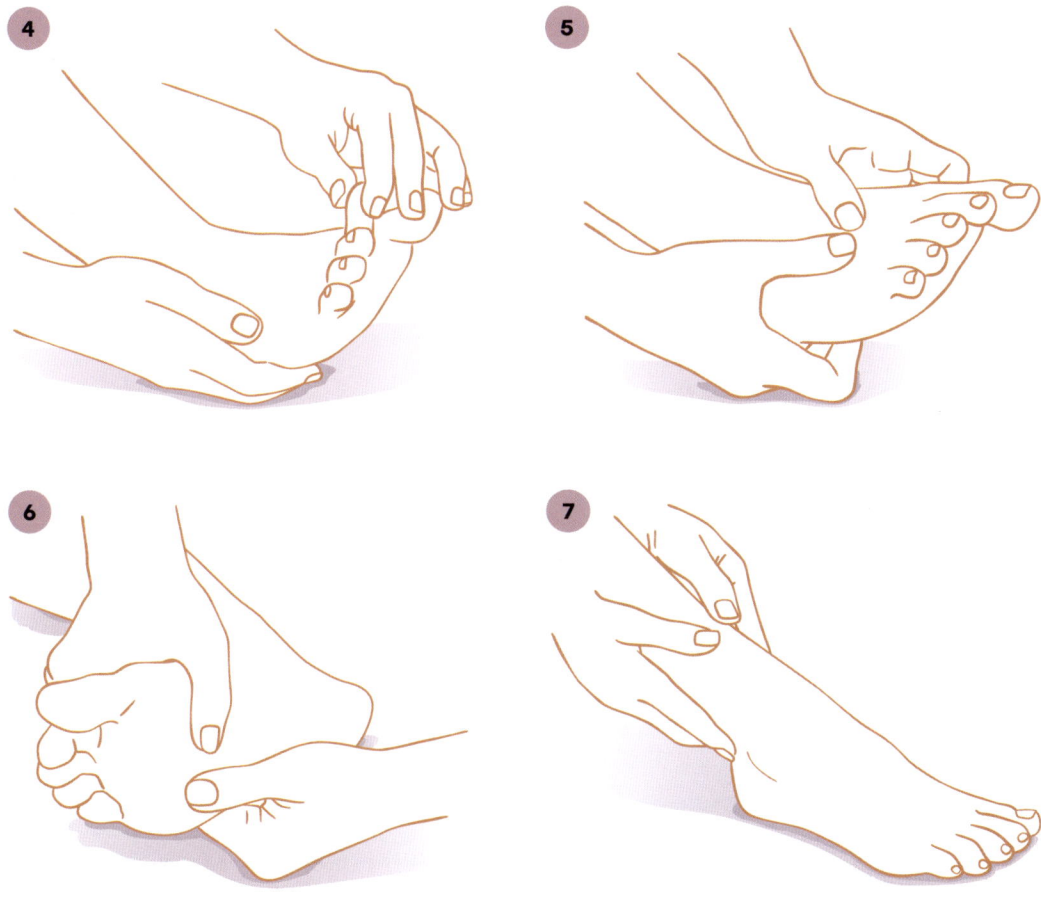

Foot care

Your feet work hard every day and really do deserve some attention, yet they are often one of the most neglected parts of the body. Regular foot care and a little TLC can make any walk far more comfortable. In fact, your foot health plays a crucial role in your overall wellbeing, independence, and quality of life.

YOU WILL NEED

- bowl of warm water
- nail clippers or scissors
- nail file
- pumice stone
- body moisturizer or foot cream
- epsom salts or tea tree oil
- cuticle cream or oil
- orange stick
- towels
- thin cotton socks

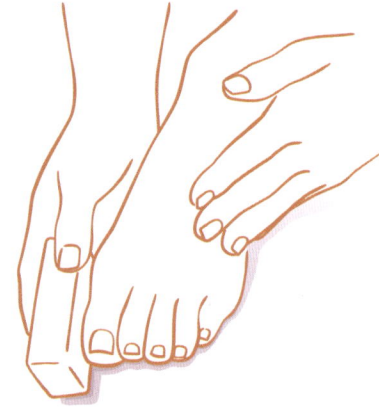

1. Make sure your feet are dry, then use a pumice stone or foot scrub to gently remove any rough or hard skin. This commonly forms on the heels, the ball of the foot, or the sides of the toes. If left to build up, hard skin can create friction between your socks and shoes during walking, leading to blisters and other irritations.

2. Once all the hard or dry skin is removed, soak your feet in a bowl of warm water for 5–10 minutes. Adding Epsom salts or a few drops of tea tree oil can help to relieve aches and pains, treat minor infections, promote relaxation, and leave your feet feeling soft and refreshed.

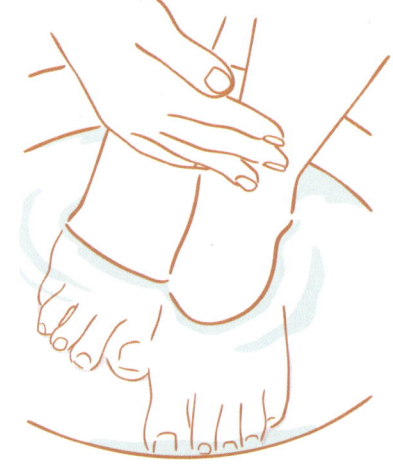

3. Thoroughly dry your feet, paying special attention to the areas between your toes. If you regularly walk, keeping your nails short will be more comfortable. Long nails can repeatedly press against the toe box as you walk, potentially causing bruising or blackened nails. Trim your toenails straight across, rounding and smoothing the edges with a nail file. This will prevent the corners from rubbing against your other toes and causing discomfort.

4. The cuticle can easily become dry or cracked. Massaging cuticle cream or oil onto this area helps keep it soft and healthy. Use an orange stick to gently push the cuticles back as trimming can encourage excessive regrowth.

5. To finish, treat yourself to a relaxing foot massage. If you're short of time, generously apply a rich body moisturizer or foot cream to your feet instead. For best results, wear cotton socks afterwards to help the cream absorb and prevent slipping.

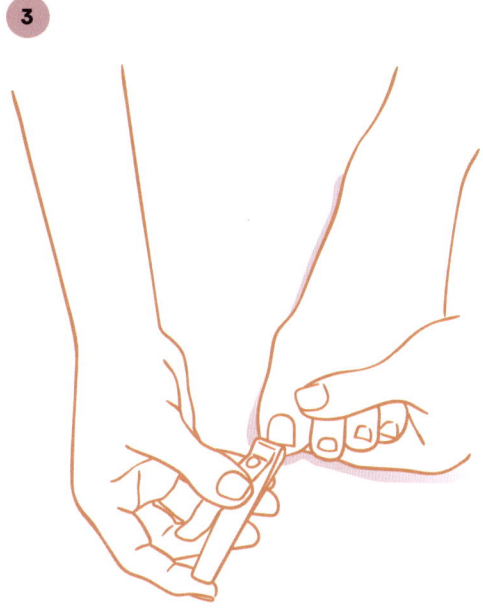

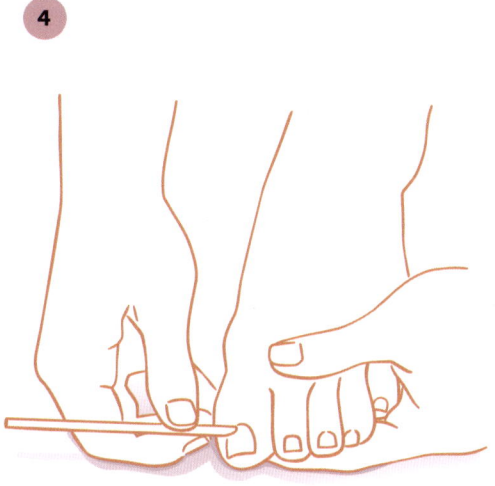

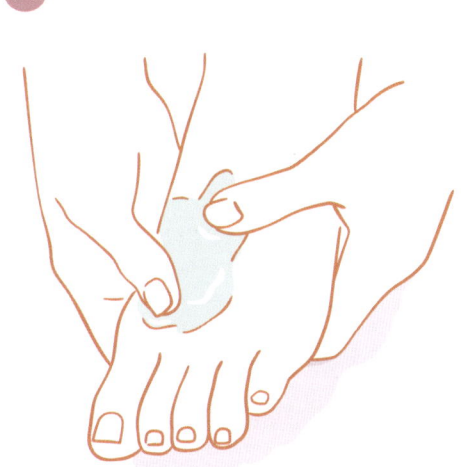

The importance of water

The human body can survive without food for weeks – even months – but without water, we would die within days. Our bodies are made up of between 65 and 70 per cent water, though that rises in very physically active people, such as athletes. The amount we drink is crucial to our health – yet many of us regularly don't drink enough.

Statistics show that as many as one person in four does not drink enough water and is dehydrated. We lose around 3 litres (5¼ pints) a day through our urine, faeces, skin, and breath, and although we absorb some water through our food, we need to drink 1.5–2 litres (2½–3½ pints) a day to replenish that loss. Many of us drink tea, coffee, or caffeinated fizzy drinks to satisfy our thirst, but too many of these have a diuretic effect instead, apart from being bad for our health. One study has shown that six cups of coffee a day causes a 3 per cent loss of water from the body.

Keeping your body well hydrated will help to regulate your body temperature and balance your electrolytes. It supports your digestion, flushes out toxins, and improves energy levels and physical performance. It will also help with mental clarity and keep your skin looking more youthful.

ARE YOU DRINKING ENOUGH?

When we are being active, or in hot weather, our bodies keep cool by sweating; during any intense activity such as a football or tennis, we can lose more than 2 litres (3.5 pints) of fluid an hour, as well as essential body salts, such as sodium, potassium, calcium bicarbonate, and phosphate. The same applies when you are exerting energy by fast walking or rucking for example; you must remember to increase your intake of fluids. Some experts in sports medicine believe that it is a mistake to use thirst as your guide, and that by the time you actually feel thirsty you are already dehydrated. Other symptoms of dehydration are irritability and a lack of concentration. Two signs that you are drinking enough water are if you urinate regularly and your urine is a very pale straw colour. Make sure you are properly hydrated before you begin walking.

KNOW YOUR WATER

Drinking water is essential to maintain good health, and it is better to drink water from any source than not at all, but not all waters are of the same quality. The purer the source of water, the more you will benefit from it.

Filtered tap water
Filtering water with activated carbon granules, whether in your tap or a filter jug, can effectively remove chemical contaminants, heavy metals, harmful pathogens, and physical particles, and prevent the presence of bacteria and germs. It also improves the taste and smell of tap water. Use your own reusable water bottle and drink filtered water when possible. A steel bottle with insulation will keep the water nice and cold.

Purified water
The most effective means of purifying water is by an undersink reverse osmosis system, which removes about 99.9 per cent of contaminants in water, including chlorine, fluoride, nitrates, and lead. The most efficient systems combine activated carbon filtration with the semi-permeable reverse osmosis membrane.

Bottled waters
Environmentally, bottled water is not a good option. However, there are times when there may be no other choice. Be selective – always read the label to identify the water source. In the USA, if the label on the bottle states "from a municipal source" or "from a community water system", you can be sure it is simply tap water. As for the bottle, opt for bottles that are recyclable, or better still choose glass bottles, as plastic can leach chemicals into the water.

Mineral water
If you do drink bottled water, this is thought to be the best choice. It is natural and untreated, and must come from an officially registered source. By law, the label must show the mineral content of the water.

Spring water
The content of spring water varies from country to country, and in some cases it is a mixture of natural and treated water. Be aware that some bottled waters are very high in sodium and inorganic minerals such as sulphates or potassium, which in this form are not easily assimilated into the body.

Carbonated water
This can be any water with carbon dioxide gas added under pressure, emulating sparkling mineral water. The carbon dioxide inhibits the growth of bacteria, and it is best without added flavours, sugars, or sweeteners that can be detrimental to teeth.

Oxygenated water
This is water to which oxygen has been added. The promise is that this will supply the muscles with more oxygen, thereby enhancing performance. However, there is currently little scientific evidence to support this claim.

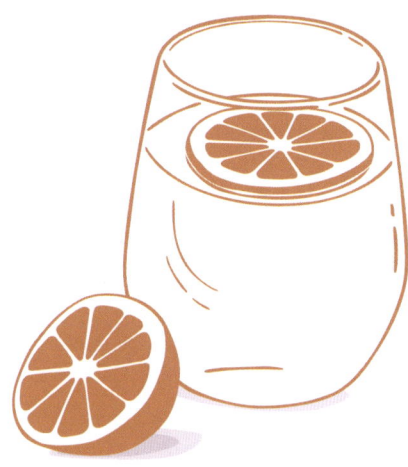

TIP In need of a change from plain water? Try adding a slice of lemon, lime, or mint to your cup or flask of hot water for a great start to your day. Or allow it to chill for a refreshing drink. On cold days, add a small slice of raw, peeled ginger to hot water. You can then just keep topping up with more hot water throughout the day: a comforting drink to take on any walk.

CARING FOR YOUR MIND AND BODY

Healthy choices

As your body grows more vital from regular walking, you will want to nourish it with food that gives you the energy you need. Consuming calorie-high, nutrient-low junk food will begin to seem less attractive, as will diets that promise speedy weight loss in exchange for cutting down on the fruit, vegetables, and carbohydrates that your body needs.

It often seems that being healthy is associated with depriving ourselves of the foods we love, but in fact good nutrition is a matter of becoming aware of what we are eating and making choices. Getting to grips with a healthier diet is very simple. Ask yourself two key questions: "Did it once have roots in soil?" and "What happened to your food before it reached you?"

FOODS WITH ROOTS
Without doubt, the very best and most nutritious of all our foods are those that started life with roots; they are full of phytochemicals and micronutrients that not only supply our bodies with everything they need, but are also easier to digest and absorb than any other foods. Every time you eat, whether it is beans on toast, curry, or Sunday lunch, always make sure that at least two-thirds of the food on your plate started life with roots in soil.

If the goal is to maximize the amount of plant-based foods that you eat, then it is also to reduce the foods that do not have roots, such as meat, dairy products, and saturated fats. The latter are normally of animal origin and tend to stay solid at room temperature. Eating too much saturated fat raises cholesterol levels in the blood, and can increase the risk of coronary heart disease, strokes, and various cancers. You should also avoid partially hydrogenated and hydrogenated vegetable oils found in hard and semi-soft margarines. These highly processed fats contain synthetic saturated fats known as trans fatty acids, which have also been linked to heart disease. Many products contain hydrogenated fats, including bread, cakes, biscuits, ready-made meals, and even chips and doughnuts from fast food outlets.

Some fats are healthy, some unhealthy, but nevertheless, our bodies need fats to help in the absorption of vitamins, and to give us essential fatty acids (EFAs). These polyunsaturated and monounsaturated fats are derived from plants, as well as the omega-3, -6, and -9 fatty acids. Omega-3, important for heart, brain, and metabolism, comes from fish, flaxseeds or flaxseed oil, and nuts such as walnuts. Omega-6 fats provide your body with energy, and are found in many different oils, seeds, tofu, and eggs. Omega-9 are nonessential fats and found in avocados, olive oil, almonds, and cashews, and a little is created by the body. Eating the right balance of this family of omega fats is vitally important for your overall health, so it is worth taking nutritional advice on achieving this balance to reach a level that supports your health and lifestyle.

THINK ABOUT WHAT YOU BUY

When it comes to buying food, what we get is often a lot more than we can see. For example, wheat is sprayed with fertilizers and other chemicals many times, and then, unwashed, is made into our bread. Our humble lettuce looks harmless, but it can be contaminated with a cocktail of artificial chemicals. Become an avid label reader and know what you are buying – ready-prepared foods that are so handy when we come home tired from work are often high in salt, preservatives, and other additives. Wherever possible, buy organic or clean food and ingredients that you can prepare in your own kitchen. Substitute refined products such as white flour, rice, and pasta with wholegrain versions.

AIM FOR THE BEST

It is unrealistic to imagine that because you decide to change your diet you will never succumb to another chocolate or fried breakfast. My philosophy is to be selective when you have these treats, and make informed choices. If you eat chocolate, eat the best organic chocolate, and if you have a fried breakfast, use the best ingredients, with unrefined oil. Treat coffee in the same way. Use freshly ground organic coffee beans, and savour each sip. This may mean foregoing your regular brew from the coffee machine at work, but if this means you drink less coffee, all the better. Make it a rule to yourself to have the best to be your best.

> "Make it a rule to yourself to have the best to be your best."

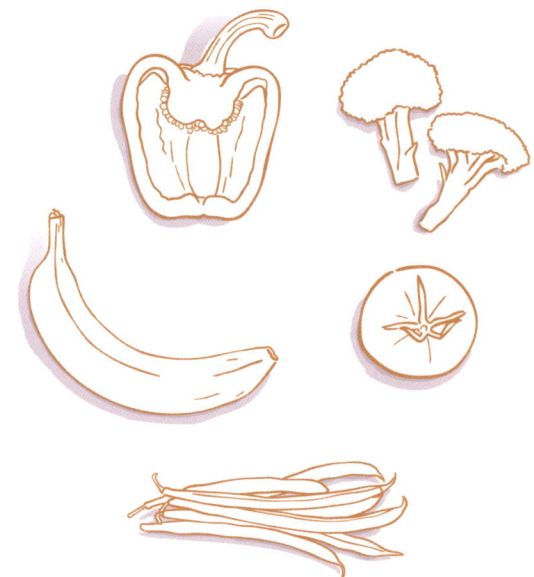

EATING OUR FIVE PORTIONS

Experts now agree that eating the minimum of five portions of vegetable and fruits a day considerably lowers the risk of heart disease or stroke by 12 per cent, and cancer by 10 per cent, with vegetables seeming to give more protection than fruit. But what equals a portion? A portion is approximately 80g (3oz). The following are some useful examples of what constitutes one serving:

- 1 medium apple
- 1 medium banana
- 150ml (5oz) fruit or vegetable juice or smoothie
- 2–3 medium carrots
- 2 heaped handfuls of lettuce
- 1 large tomato or 5 cherry tomatoes
- 5–6 florets of broccoli
- ½ a large courgette
- ½ a pepper
- 80g (3oz) of beans or other pulses

CARING FOR YOUR MIND AND BODY

Vitamins and minerals

Other than vitamin D, we can only get the vitamins, minerals, and micronutrients we need from our food. There is plenty of evidence to show that eating well provides the energy to live life at your healthy best, as well as reducing your risk of disease, but putting it into practice can be quite overwhelming to begin with.

Eating a rainbow of fruits and vegetables is a really good place to start. Each plant contains different colour pigments or phytonutrients, which have been linked to specific health benefits. Red fruits and vegetables, such as tomatoes and peppers, contain lycopene, and become even more effective when cooked. They are a powerful antioxidant, thought to protect against cancer. Orange and yellow, such as citrus fruits, carrots, or bananas, contain carotenoids, which are rich antioxidants; good for eye health and boosting the immune system.

Green fruits and vegetables including kale, spinach, broccoli, kiwi, and avocados are high in vitamin K and can help to maintain strong teeth and bones as well as protect against cancer. Blues and purples – aubergines, blueberries, grapes, and plums – contain anthocyanins and antioxidants associated with brain health and memory. Dark red fruits and vegetables such as beetroot contain betalains, thought to help your heart and lungs work better during exercise.

Vitamins cannot be assimilated into the body without minerals. Together these two vital substances, along with carbohydrates, proteins, fats, and water, provide you with the essential nutrients for cell growth, tissue repair, organ function, energy, and food utilization.

NATURAL SUPPLEMENTS

Organic foods fresh from your local area is ideal. Unfortunately, many of the foods grown today have very depleted vitamin and almost no mineral content. This is because of intensive farming practices, as well as transportation and storage methods – even when our intake of nutrients is sufficient, factors such stress, taking medications, smoking, or living in a polluted atmosphere all take their toll. Opinions vary as to whether or not taking nutritional supplements is useful, but my own view is that they contributed to my recovery from cancer. A good-quality multivitamin, a dose of vitamin C, and vitamin D is now universally recommended for most people, but it is advisable to visit a nutritionist for advice or carry out some research into your own requirements first. Buy the best-quality supplements you can afford – check the ingredients for the quantity in each dose, and also for the quality. Make sure that the ingredients are from natural sources. Avoid synthetic vitamins, which can cause toxic reactions and can contribute to poor health.

THE JOY OF JUICING

Raw fruits and vegetables that have been juiced retain vitamins and enzymes that are often destroyed in the cooking process. Juicing machines and juicing attachments for food processors are now widely available. As a guide, the better the machine, the better the results, especially with root vegetables.

WHERE TO FIND SOME OF YOUR MOST IMPORTANT VITAMINS AND MINERALS

Vitamin A	Apricots, cabbage, carrots, curly kale, egg yolks, fish-liver oil (from an uncontaminated source), mango, melon, spinach, squash, sweet potato, Swiss chard, yellow peppers, watercress
Vitamin B group:	
B1 *(thiamine)*	Beans, bran, most vegetables, whole grains, yeast
B2 *(riboflavin)*	Eggs, leafy green vegetables, mushrooms, tomatoes, wheatgerm
B3 *(niacin)*	Cabbage, cauliflower, mushrooms, tomatoes
B5 *(pantothenic acid)*	Alfalfa sprouts, avocados, broccoli, cabbage, celery, eggs, lentils, mushrooms, squash, tomatoes
B6	Bananas, broccoli, Brussels sprouts, cabbage, cauliflower, lentils, nuts, onions, squash
B12	Eggs
Vitamin C	Citrus fruits, broccoli, cabbage, cauliflower, kiwi fruit, melon, papaya, peas, peppers, sprouted seeds, strawberries, tomatoes
Vitamin D and K	Egg yolk
Vitamin E	Beans, broccoli, raw leafy green vegetables, peas, pine nuts, sunflower and sesame seeds, unrefined corn oils, wheatgerm, wholegrain cereals
Folic acid	Avocados, broccoli, cashew nuts, cauliflower, hazelnuts, spinach, walnuts, wheatgerm
Calcium	Almonds, brewer's yeast, cabbage, dried beans, green vegetables, nuts, sunflower seeds
Iron	Dates, dried beans, egg yolks, miso, nuts, oats, pumpkin and sesame seeds
Selenium	Brazil nuts, broccoli, cabbage, courgettes, haricot beans, lentils, mushrooms, wheatgerm
Zinc	Almonds, Brazil nuts, brewer's yeast, egg yolks, oats, pumpkin seeds, rye, wholewheat

Foods for health and fitness

When you are exercising regularly, your diet will help your body to perform at its best. Exercise burns up energy in our bodies, and to achieve best results you need to ensure that you have enough fuel to sustain that energy. Physical activity without eating the right foods is like putting your foot down on the accelerator and suddenly finding you have no power.

Nourishing yourself with the right foods to provide energy becomes even more essential when you increase the physical demands on your body. Carbohydrates, such as whole grains, beans, and lentils, provide a constant source of energy. Proteins, found in eggs, oily fish, lean meat, and nuts are essential for building bones and repairing tissue. It is also important to stay hydrated; everyone should drink a minimum of 6–8 glasses of water a day, more if you are being active.

CARBOHYDRATES

The best fuel for sustained exercise is carbohydrates, which are broken down to glucose in the body and stored primarily in your muscles and liver as glycogen. This is then converted back into glucose to provide energy for the muscles you are exercising. The body can only store a certain amount of glycogen, which cannot be transferred from resting muscles to those that are working. As you walk, your muscles can become quickly depleted. Consequently, it is important to keep your levels topped up, and to have a carbohydrate snack immediately after exercise to speed recovery.

Although all carbohydrates are converted to glucose in the body, the rate at which they are absorbed differs widely. Foods such as beans, legumes, and whole grains are absorbed slowly and will provide fuel over the longer term, making them ideal foods if you are going to undertake strenuous exercise.

A PLANT-BASED DIET

Studies have consistently shown that people who eat a vegetarian diet live longer than meat eaters and have lower incidences of many major diseases, including cancer, heart disease, and diabetes. Yet many people have concerns about meeting all their nutritional needs through a vegetarian diet, especially when they are active in sports. It is sometimes thought, for example, that an athlete needs to tuck into a large steak to gain sufficient protein, but this is not necessary. We can in fact obtain all the proteins we need from many plant foods, including soya, pulses, grains, and all nuts and seeds. A word of warning though: do not replace meat with equivalent amounts of cheese since it is high in saturated fats.

Eating a wide range of plant-based foods will provide you with a high intake of antioxidants and phytochemicals, all of which have innumerable health-giving properties. They will also provide a good source of calcium (found in, for example, raw broccoli, sunflower seeds, almonds, and Brazil nuts), which is vital for strong, healthy bones and keeping active.

LONG-DISTANCE WALKING

Your diet and hydration play an important part in providing you with energy and sustainability for long walks. This applies during preparation, but also during the challenge, and the recovery.

The week before
Keep your food light, simple, and easy to digest. Eat plenty of vegetables, and include one vegetable juice or smoothie a day. Salads with light dressings, grilled fish (or very lean meat), and plenty of unrefined carbohydrates such as potatoes, rice, or quinoa. Avoid rich, spicy dishes, fried foods, and big meals that are heavy to digest. Eat every 2–3 hours, as well as regular snacks such as a peanut butter sandwich, or a bagel. Also remembering to continue to keep well hydrated.

The day before
Have two high-carbohydrate meals. Always try to eat your largest meal in the middle of the day, so that your body does not have to work hard at digestion through the night.

The Big Day and the recovery
Eat a hot meal 1–2 hours before setting off – it may be the last hot sustenance you have for many hours. Include a mix of carbohydrates and proteins that slowly release energy throughout the day. Consider foods such as eggs, grilled chicken, brown rice and vegetables, whole grains, or yogurt with a fruit smoothie. Caffeine can help performance, but remember tea and coffee are both diuretic. For high-intensity walking, apart from regularly sipping water, keep replenishing your energy levels every 1–2 hours with foods such as bananas, raisins, or a low-fat granola bar. Within 30 minutes of completing your challenge, eat energy-giving foods, as this is when your body is most effective at converting carbohydrates into the much needed glycogen. Within 2 hours of finishing, eat a full meal including all macronutrients to speed up recovery.

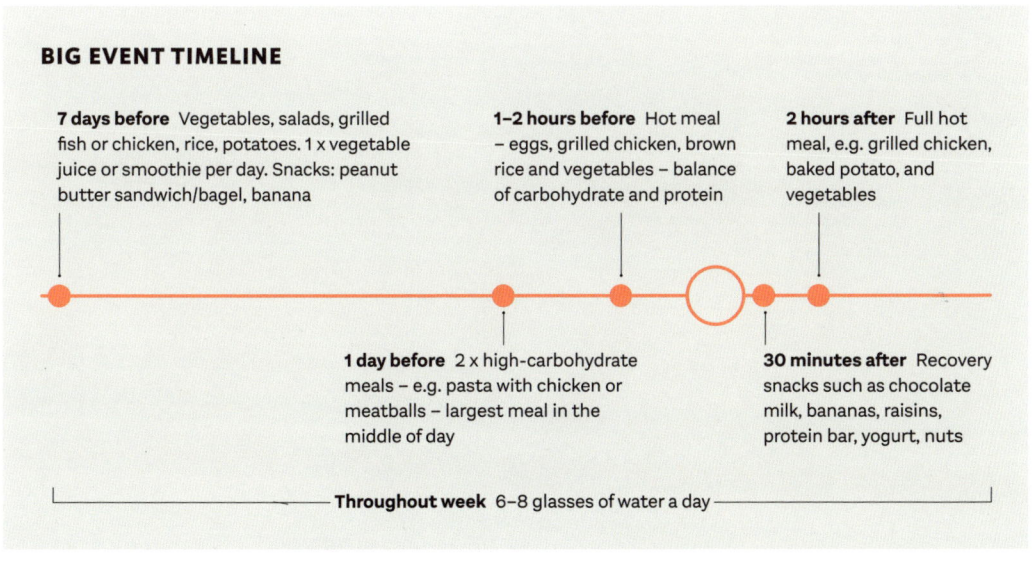

BIG EVENT TIMELINE

7 days before Vegetables, salads, grilled fish or chicken, rice, potatoes. 1 x vegetable juice or smoothie per day. Snacks: peanut butter sandwich/bagel, banana

1 day before 2 x high-carbohydrate meals – e.g. pasta with chicken or meatballs – largest meal in the middle of day

1–2 hours before Hot meal – eggs, grilled chicken, brown rice and vegetables – balance of carbohydrate and protein

30 minutes after Recovery snacks such as chocolate milk, bananas, raisins, protein bar, yogurt, nuts

2 hours after Full hot meal, e.g. grilled chicken, baked potato, and vegetables

Throughout week 6–8 glasses of water a day

ENERGY-BOOSTING FOODS

Bananas One of the richest sources of potassium, which helps to regulate muscle contractions. Bananas replenish the potassium lost through sweating – an ideal snack on the go!

Brown rice A complex carbohydrate with twice the fibre and nutrients of white rice. It is the best rice for slow absorption. As well as being a good source of protein, it also contains zinc, magnesium, vitamin B6, and selenium.

Pasta Choose wholewheat or buckwheat pasta when you are looking for slow-burning fuel for your muscles. A pasta dish is the perfect pre-marathon meal. Pasta also provides iron, and the B vitamins thiamine, niacin, and riboflavin.

Broccoli High in fibre, a good source of iron and folic acid. Iron helps to bind oxygen in red blood cells, which is then transported and used by the body's muscles, organs, and tissues. Folic acid is important for the health of red blood cells and keeping cholesterol levels under control. If eaten raw, broccoli also provides calcium.

Beans and legumes Superb slow-burning foods that are also high in protein and are a good source of folic acid (see Broccoli, below).

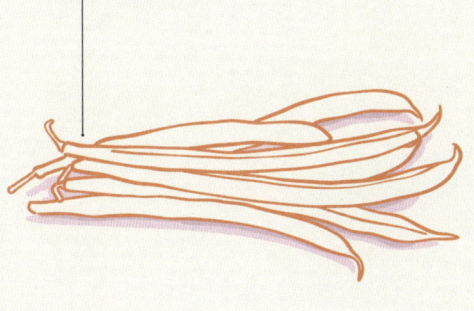

Carrot juice When freshly juiced (see p115) it is a concentrated source of vitamin A (beta carotene), which is essential for the growth and repair of body tissues, and will help to fight infections.

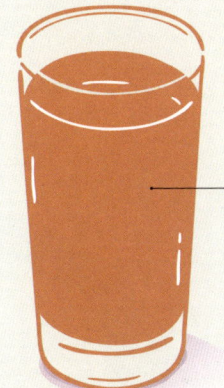

Dried fruits An excellent concentrated source of energy and rich in iron and calcium. They are high in fructose and very sweet, but they make a good snack to bring with you on your walk.

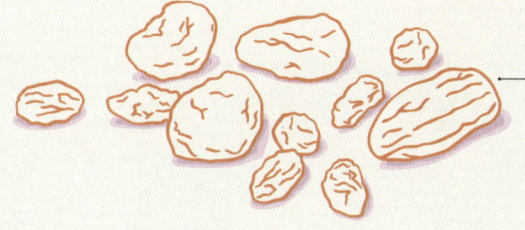

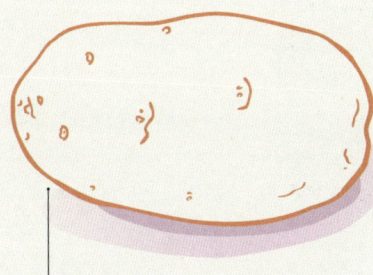

Potatoes A medium-sized portion provides twice the potassium of a banana and is high in vitamin C and iron. Excellent for boosting blood energy levels and fighting fatigue.

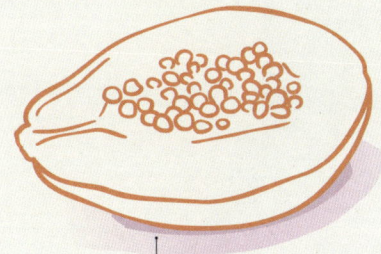

Papaya Has as much potassium as bananas (see opposite), as well as high levels of vitamin C and beta carotene (see Carrot juice, above).

CARING FOR YOUR MIND AND BODY

6

Ways to walk

Exploring different types of walking will not only offer physical challenges, but also add enough variety to keep you motivated on every walk. Try combining road walking with trail walking and include other types of terrain for some of your walks. Rucking and Nordic walking are other ways to change up your routine.

Road walking

Country roads or busy urban streets offer accessibility and provide smooth, flat surfaces that are easy to walk on. While you need to be mindful about road safety, road walking is ideal if you prefer walking on even ground, or want to pick up the pace and increase the intensity of your walking workout.

If you're preparing for a long-distance walk, training for a fast-paced walk like a marathon, or simply aiming to boost your fitness, tarmac and pavement offer an ideal opportunity to work on speed and try interval walking. Interval training can be applied to any type of walking or activity, from road racing to rucking, but is best approached on a flat surface. Only begin when you have reached a basic cardiovascular fitness level (see pp8–9).

HOW TO BEGIN INTERVAL TRAINING

Set a cycle that includes brief intervals of walking at a high intensity, which increases your heart rate to an aerobic level and boosts oxygen flow to your muscles and back to your lungs. Follow this with a period of lower-intensity activity for anaerobic recovery. In this process, your body switches from using oxygen to stored carbohydrate energy.

The ratio between the high-intensity activity, and the slower recovery pace, should depend on your level of fitness. As a guide, start with a 1:2 ratio: for every 1 minute walked at an intense, fast pace, double the time for the slow, recovery pace. If it feels too tough or too easy, adjust the length of intervals accordingly. To begin with, the slower-speed intervals should be longer, lasting from 2–15 minutes. As your fitness improves, try a 1:1 ratio, so that the periods of fast and slow walking are equal in length. Use a heart-rate monitor to keep a check on how hard you are working (see p9 and p53). Depending on your age, do not exceed 80–95 per cent of your maximum heart rate during the high intensity phase.

First steps: Begin as you would for any walk – find your regular pace, and then start your session (see pp60–67). The periods of high-intensity walking should feel like all-out exertion, while the slower periods are to recover your breath, preparing you to repeat the cycle again. The aim is to keep intervals constant and steady, so ensure you don't start with a pace that you can't maintain for every round. Complete as many sets as you can within 30 minutes and then end your session as normal (see pp90–95). This time can increase as your fitness improves.

A powerful combination: Alternating between high and low intensities is not easy, but it is a powerful combination that can greatly benefit your overall fitness and health. Working at an aerobic level will help you to develop your strength and stamina, as well as promote good heart health, prevent diabetes, and reduce anxiety. Exercising anaerobically can also promote strong bone density, build muscle, and burn fat.

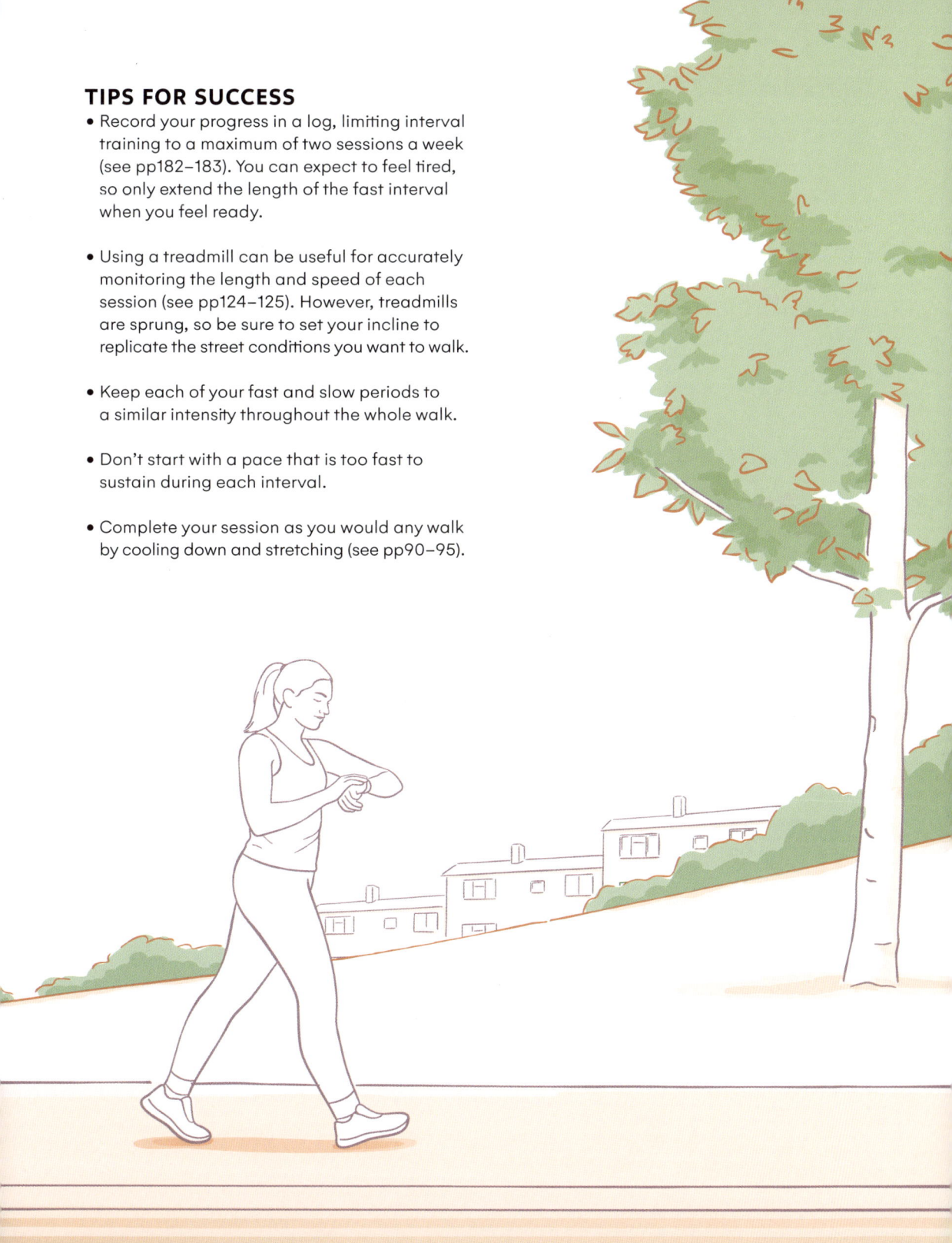

TIPS FOR SUCCESS

- Record your progress in a log, limiting interval training to a maximum of two sessions a week (see pp182–183). You can expect to feel tired, so only extend the length of the fast interval when you feel ready.

- Using a treadmill can be useful for accurately monitoring the length and speed of each session (see pp124–125). However, treadmills are sprung, so be sure to set your incline to replicate the street conditions you want to walk.

- Keep each of your fast and slow periods to a similar intensity throughout the whole walk.

- Don't start with a pace that is too fast to sustain during each interval.

- Complete your session as you would any walk by cooling down and stretching (see pp90–95).

Treadmill walking

A treadmill will never replace the experience of walking outside, but don't dismiss it too soon. It is a versatile piece of equipment with many benefits. It provides a consistent surface on which to develop technique, gives accurate calculations for interval walking, and allows you to set your own incline. You also won't need to worry about the weather!

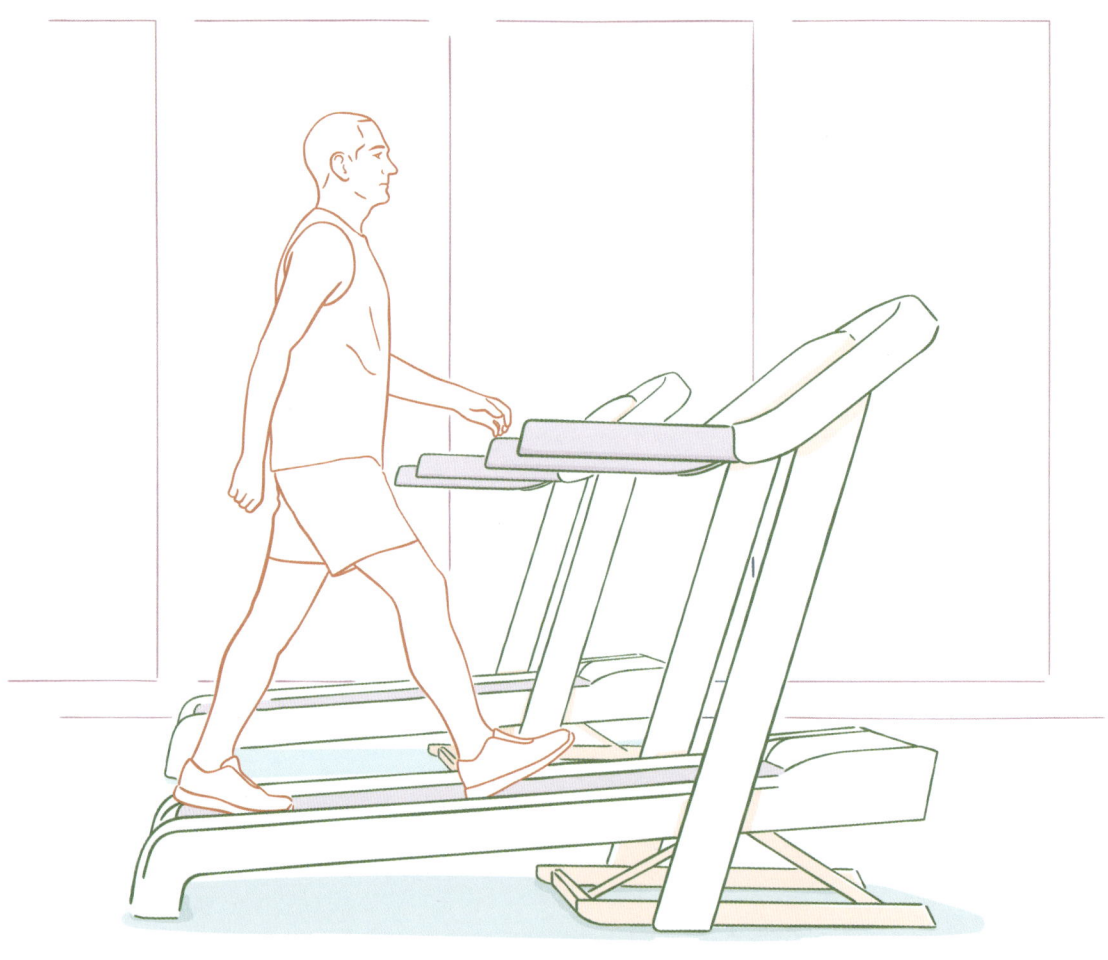

BENEFITS OF A TREADMILL

Due to the moving belt that simulates a road, treadmills offer low-impact, low-risk workout for walking or running. You're in complete control of a versatile range of programmes that can be set to suit you and your fitness plan. In this controlled environment, where there's no excuse not to walk, it not only helps keep you active but also supports your mental wellbeing and motivation to keep going.

THE IMPORTANCE OF AN INCLINE

The experience of walking on a treadmill is very different from walking on a road. Due to the cushioning of the belt, the impact is softer, making walking, jogging, or running easier and faster, and placing less strain on your joints. Get to know your treadmill functions and what it is capable of. To compensate for the softer surface, even if you are a beginner, it is important to check that the treadmill is set to an incline of 1 per cent, which will replicate conditions on a road, encouraging you to use the same level of exertion. With some machines you can even switch the cushioning on and off.

MONITORING AND STRETCHING

Including the use of a heart-rate monitor is an effective way to assess your fitness, and to improve the quality of your workout. Most people use their watch or smartphone (see pp52–53). Entry level machines may have built-in hand grip monitors, while more advanced treadmills will include Bluetooth-enabled chest straps or arm bands. Preparing for a session should include stretching and good posture, the same as any other walk (see pp60–61 and pp90–91). However, never stretch while on the treadmill or walk barefoot, and always be cautious with the speed. Set the pace within your ability, only increasing it in small increments when you are ready, to avoid stress on your shins, or losing balance.

CUSTOMIZING YOUR WORKOUTS

The fun part of walking on a treadmill is customizing and creating your workouts. Set your goals and how long you want the session to last. Whether you want to take on a high-intensity challenge, follow a speed program, work on technique, or conquer mountain inclines, remember that you have access to it all. Keep your workouts varied: slow and steady wins the race. If you think it might be boring, try testing your coordination by walking backwards, holding onto the rails if necessary, or using light weights or a rucking jacket. Workout to music, walk while watching your favourite TV show, or try out an under-desk treadmill that will allow you to work while you walk; it will all contribute to your overall health and fitness, and make you a stronger walker.

WALKING PADS

Unlike conventional treadmills, under-desk treadmills are compact – some are even foldable – and will fit comfortably under a desk. Many have a built-in screen at the top to show walking metrics. You'll need a height-adjustable or standing desk to use it comfortably. You could also move it to the TV room and walk while watching your favourite shows.

Hiking

Hiking, trail walking, or trekking – travelling over uneven terrain and conquering the ups and downs of hills – is a great way to strengthen your leg and core muscles, while also testing your endurance and stability. Venturing off the beaten track with everything you need on your back brings a great sense of freedom, no matter how long it is for.

Hiking can be as physically demanding as you want it to be. Often it is the hills or unexpected challenging terrain where the enjoyment lies. But all hiking needs careful preparation. You need to take into account how far you intend to travel, the ground conditions, your ability, what you wear, and what you take with you. Just like road walking, start small with short, manageable distances that give your body time to adjust to changes in your stride, breathing, and walking up and down different gradients.

CHANGES IN YOUR TECHNIQUE

Aim to maintain a consistent pace from the beginning of your hike to the end by finding a rhythm that connects your breathing to your pace and stride, while being mindful that this may change depending on the terrain. Your ability should determine the speed at which you walk, but consistency is key to preserving energy. As you start to climb, lean slightly forwards into the incline, while shortening your stride to manage the terrain. If the going does get tough as the angle becomes more acute, try repeating a mantra to keep you focused on reaching your goal (see p129). Walking downhill may feel like a reward after the climb, but it can be just as challenging for even the most experienced walkers. When you walk downhill the impact of your body weight increases from 1.5 to 5 times your normal weight. This puts extra stress on your limbs and joints. If you are using adjustable walking poles, lengthen them as you descend, to prevent leaning too far forward as you plant the poles. Make sure you use trekking, not Nordic walking poles, as the latter are geared towards a specific type of walking (see pp134–135).

Keep your stride short and lean back slightly. You may want to zigzag back and forth across the area, much like a skier, to make your way down. This reduces the angle of the gradient, puts less pressure on your toes, and gives you more control overall.

THE RIGHT SHOES FOR TERRAIN AND WEATHER

The right shoes are key to your overall comfort (see pp36–41), and should be appropriate for the type of terrain and weather conditions you are expecting. If you are going to be covering rugged or wet ground, wear a boot that offers good ankle support, deep treads on the sole for traction, and is made from Gore-Tex or similar. In warmer weather, opt for a trail shoe in a more breathable fabric. You may even find that you also need to tape your feet to protect them from blisters, especially on multiday treks and in hot climates. Before going out on a hike, get used to the weight of your footwear, feel how your socks fit, and decide which lacing works best.

CLOTHING AND USEFUL EXTRAS

On less challenging hikes, the rule of thumb is to opt for light wicking fabrics and layers (see pp46–49). Stay prepared for rapid weather changes by carrying a windproof jacket, a fleece, and waterproofs. For more extreme conditions, it's important to seek specialist advice on a more technical approach to your attire.

For shorter hikes, a well-fitting day backpack should be comfortable to wear and hold everything you need, including waterproofs, a water bottle, food or snacks, insect repellent, a spare phone battery, a torch, and a small medical kit. A compass and paper map are also good tools to carry in case of losing digital connections if you know how to use them.

Regular stretching (see Chapter 4) while on the move is essential to prevent stiffness, especially in the neck and shoulders. It's also important to take breaks (with snacks and water) little and often, to keep you going stronger for longer!

> "Conquering the ups and downs of hills is a great way to strengthen your leg and core muscles, as well as testing your endurance and stability."

Mindful walking

Meditation is often referred to as an act of mindfulness, where the mind is focused on a single point or activity in the present moment. Most people assume that to meditate you must sit cross-legged on the floor with your eyes closed, but it is just as possible, if not easier, to meditate while walking.

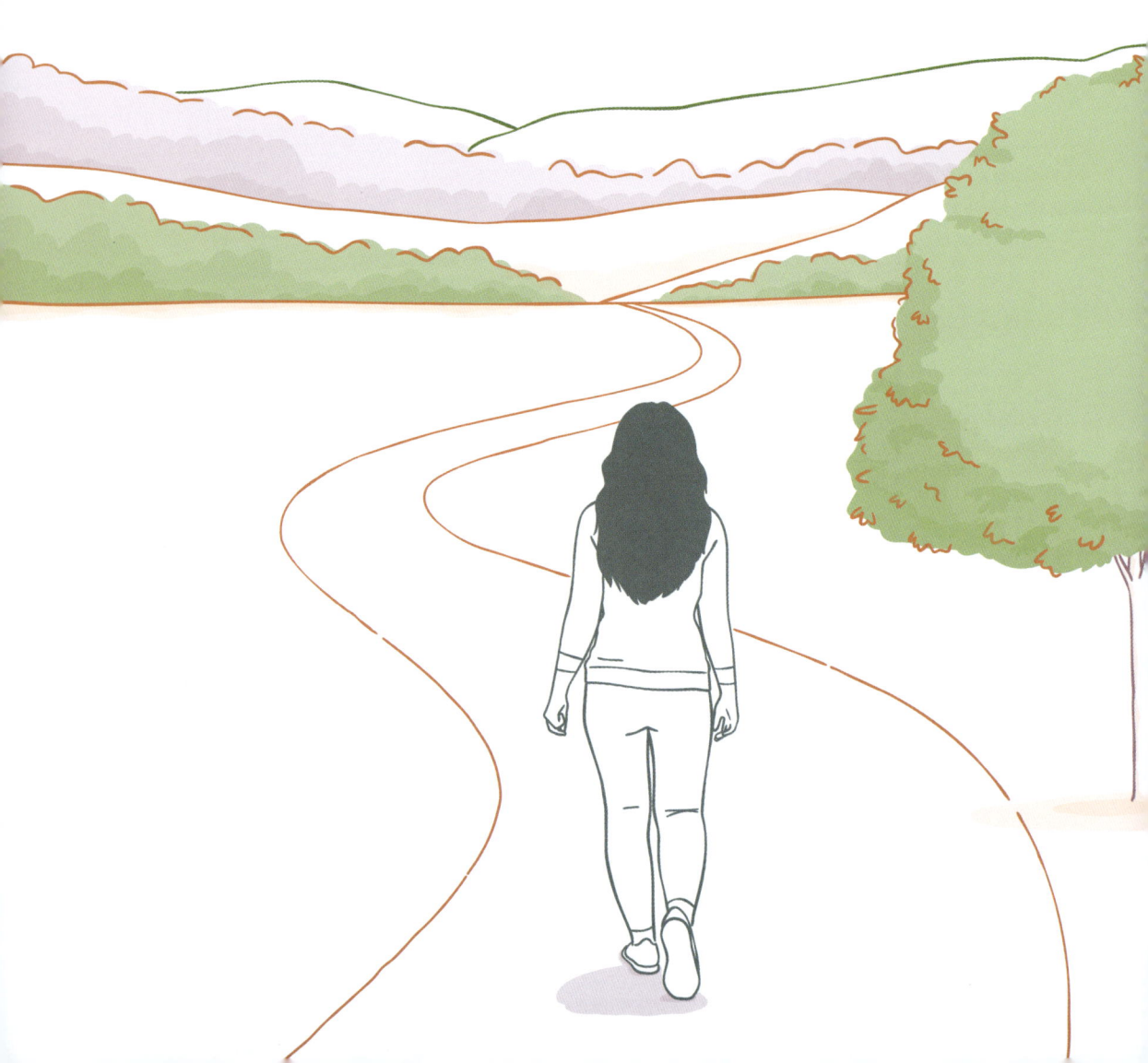

In fact, walking with awareness in the present moment is a wonderful way to spend time walking alone and can bring great emotional and physical rewards.

The benefits of practising meditation are well documented, including promoting inner balance, mental clarity, reducing stress levels, and improving sleep. Focusing on your breath and the physical rhythm of walking can create a harmonious connection between body and mind. With each step comes the opportunity to enhance your physical and mental wellbeing.

AWARENESS OF YOUR MOVEMENT

Pay close attention to your feet while you find your pace. Notice every step, and how each foot, left and right, connects to the ground as it rolls from heel to toe. Now bring your awareness to your ankles, calves, knees, and thighs. Notice how your hips lift and fall while you move, as the weight transfers with each step. Feel your belly as the centre of your being, and notice how with each breath, your lungs fill, and your chest expands. As you breathe out, relax the muscles in your shoulders and neck, allowing your chin to lift, your jaw to soften, and your head to rise. With your eyes gently focused ahead, enjoy the rhythm of meditation in motion, as your arms and legs move freely. Walk slowly, fully engaging all your senses, and staying aware of your surroundings. With a balanced head position (see pp60–61), you will feel the muscles in your neck relax and elongate. Relax your jaw and keep your eyes gently focused ahead. If something distracts you, simply notice it and return your attention to walking.

REPEATING A MANTRA

Another way to keep your mind in the present moment is to repeat a mantra. This can be a word, a group of words, or a sound that will help to keep the mind centred. Choose a mantra that feels comfortable and relevant to you, and will allow your feet to fall into a rhythmic step with each word or phrase as you repeat it. I have frequently used mantras to cope with some of the most difficult times in my life, to affirm positivity when I am taking on a challenge such as a marathon, and to promote calm and wellbeing in day-to-day life. One of my favourites is "I am fit and I am healthy." Repeat your mantra for at least 15 minutes, letting the rhythm of the words flow with each breath, filling your mind and grounding you with each step. There will be times when you will lose your concentration and busy thoughts of the day's tasks and activities will intrude, but quietly put them to one side and reconnect with your mantra. As you reach the end of your walk, end your meditation and reconnect with your surroundings. Once you have mastered mindful walking, you can do it whenever you want to feel a restored sense of balance.

Rucking

Rucking, which involves walking wearing a weighted rucksack or jacket, increases the physical intensity and impact walking already has on your body. It takes your normal walk and turns it into a full-body cardio fitness workout.

Rucking is low impact, so unlikely to cause injury, provided you work within your ability. As a cardiovascular exercise, it will increase your heart rate, as well as engaging almost all of the major muscle groups used in strength training. It can also have the very positive effects of lowering blood pressure, improving bone density, and strengthening your core. Overall, it helps build greater physical and mental resilience, as well as endurance and wellbeing, impacting all aspects of your everyday life.

HISTORY AND PRACTICE OF RUCKING

The original practice of rucking was developed for military training, but it is suitable for everyone, from families to hard-core fitness fanatics, as you can choose the weights to put into the backpack. Regular "ruckers" will use purpose-built backpacks or rucking jackets that are measured by their litre capacity. As part of the system, the pack will hold cast-iron rucking plates that go up in increments from 5–25kg (11–55lb).

Provided your existing backpack is a good fit, you can use it for rucking, adding relatively low weights. Put a kettlebell, dumbbell, or even a brick into it, and wrap it in something similar to a towel, loading it in a way that distributes the weight evenly.

GETTING STARTED

If you want to give it a go, all you need to get started is a well-fitting backpack – go light with the weight – and either boots or trail shoes depending on the time of year and terrain. It is also advisable to wear breathable and moisture wicking clothing as you will likely build up a sweat! Of course, once you get the feel of it, you may want to be more specific, and invest in your equipment.

BACKPACK CHECK LIST

☑ Any backpack should fit closely against your back and be suited to your height, shape, and weight for the best comfort and support.

☑ Wide, adjustable straps, ideally with a chest and waist strap, will help to support and distribute the load, especially as you add to it. Adjust the straps so the backpack fits snugly to your body.

☑ Take into account the additional weight you could be carrying, including a hydration bladder, which will help to keep your hands free, or a water bottle (making sure there is an external holder on the pack to carry it in).

☑ Add wet weather kit, snacks, and spare socks, if you are going to be rucking for a few days.

HOW MUCH WEIGHT?

Consider your fitness level, personal comfort, and goals when choosing weights. As a beginner, your day backpack, including water, should not weigh more than 10–15 per cent of your body weight. This level will achieve aerobic fitness and weight control. If you are wanting to build muscle and endurance, you will need to work up to 20–30 per cent of your body weight, adding weight in increments of 2.2kg–4.5kg (5lb–10lb), as your strength and stamina increase.

HOW FAR?

Plan your distance, starting from 2–5km (1–3 miles), gradually increasing as you progress. I would recommend using a training plan (see Chapter 7) to begin with so that you have some structure to track your distance and weight. If you are rucking in preparation for a long challenge, build up your weight and distance slowly. Always wear a backpack on all your training walks. You may also want to add walking poles into the mix (see p126).

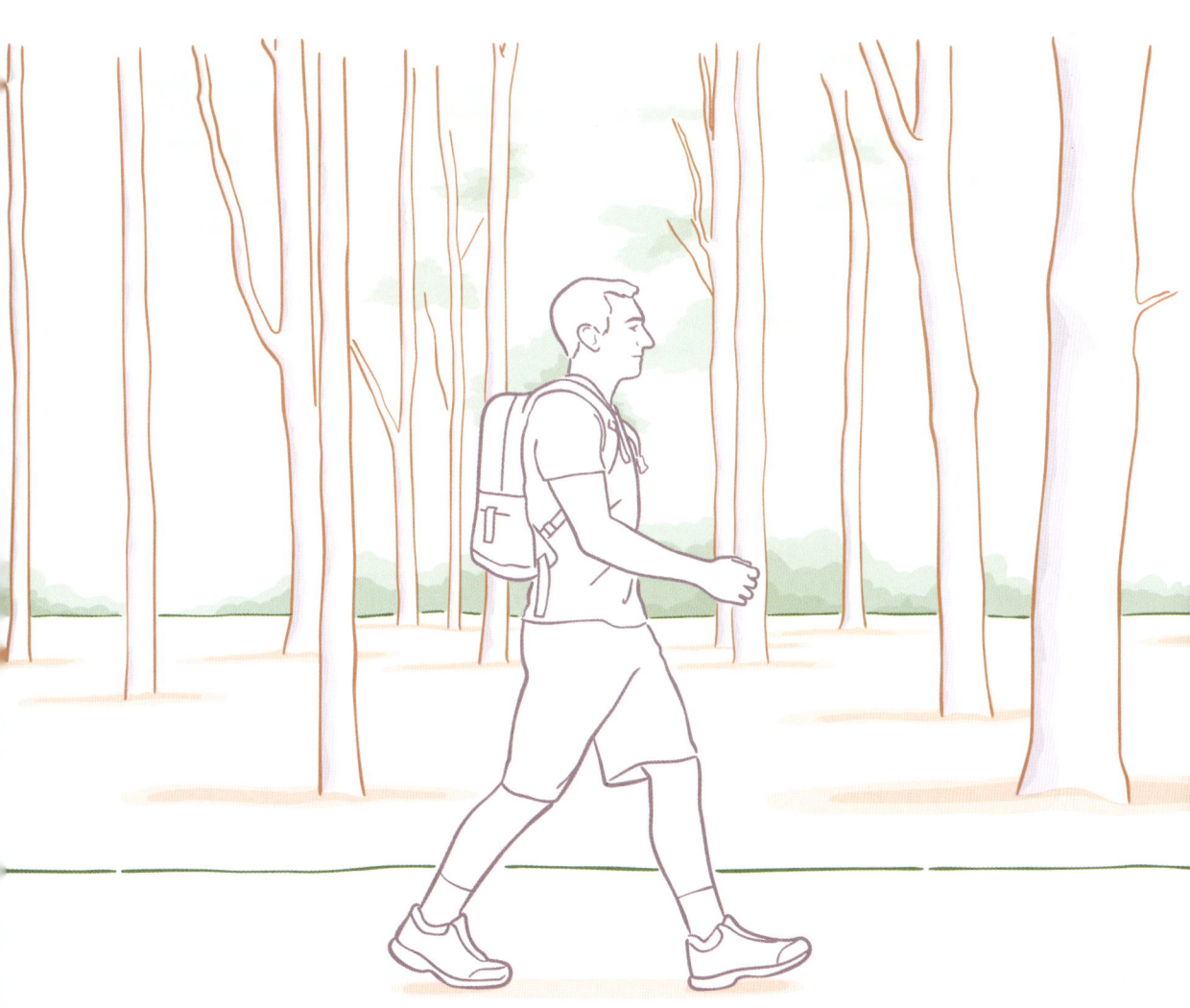

Barefoot walking

According to some orthopaedic professionals, walking barefoot helps to restore our natural walking pattern (our "gait"), while strengthening the intricate structure of the feet. The sensory nerves in the feet allow you to connect with the earth and to feel wonderful sensations you miss when wearing shoes.

Feet are complex structures – each foot is made up of more than 100 moving parts, including bones, muscles, tendons, and ligaments, as well as thousands of sensory nerves.

Don't head straight out the door barefoot – start with just 10 minutes a day at home. The technique begins with good posture (see pp60–61). It is tempting to keep your eyes fixed on the floor in case you accidently walk on something undesirable, but try to keep your eye line a few steps ahead. Use the heel to toe rolling action (see pp62–63), adapting it for bare feet by making the "heel strike" much gentler, followed by an immediate roll forward. Always lift your back foot as you bring it forward. The surface of the ground will determine whether you place your weight onto the ball, or the flat mid-sole section of your foot. It may feel exaggerated to begin with, but try to consciously use the full range of your foot.

HEADING OUTSIDE

Increase the time by 5 minutes each day. When you are ready, start venturing out into the garden. Then, in your own time, slowly widen the area you walk. Allow yourself to experience the sensations of different textures such as grassy fields and woodland paths (see "grounding", p24). Feel the resistance as your heel sinks into sand, grass, or soil. Keep your feet well moisturized to stop the skin from drying. It is a good idea to carry your shoes, so you can stop if you are uncomfortable or feel any pain.

CAUTIONS FOR BAREFOOT WALKING

Before you abandon your shoes to try barefoot walking, there are a few things to keep in mind.

- Some public areas may not be sociably acceptable, or suitable for bare feet. Always tread where you can see a clear path ahead, avoiding sharp or harmful objects. Never walk barefoot in extremes of temperature.

- The soles of your feet are three times thicker than on other parts of your body, but as we age, the pads on the balls of our feet, and underneath the heel bone, become thinner, providing less of a protective cushion.

- Also be aware of picking up fungal and bacterial infections – you increase this risk when walking barefoot in the great outdoors.

- If you have foot conditions such as collapsed arches, arthritis of the big toe, plantar fasciitis (see p45), or diabetes, wearing supportive cushioned footwear is essential.

MINIMALIST SHOES

If you like the idea, but walking completely barefoot is a step too far, try minimalist shoes. They have no arch support, heel rise, and a very wide toe box. They are as close as you can get to replicating the sensation of being barefoot, while wearing a shoe. While not recommended as your go-to daily footwear, for many, they are the ideal sports shoe. Whether you go barefoot, or opt for minimalist shoes, it is important to first understand your feet (see pp36–37) and that along with the benefits, there are also risks.

FINDING COMPANY

If you're looking for some like-minded enthusiasts, there are barefoot clubs and organizations across the globe, and you can also use apps to find out about trails and treks that are suitably rated for barefoot hikers. Whatever your view, it should never take away the pleasure of connecting with nature, by just taking your shoes off, and feeling the healing earth beneath your feet.

"Allow yourself to experience the sensations of different textures such as grassy fields and woodland paths."

Nordic walking

Originating in Finland, Nordic walking is a technique very similar in action to cross-country skiing. Walking with poles engages the upper body and allows a longer stride as you move forward. It is not only a great way to add variety to your walking repertoire, it has also been proven to have a number of direct health benefits.

BENEFITS OF NORDIC WALKING

- It can increase your exercise capacity and oxygen intake, while also improving blood circulation and heart health.

- Walking with poles helps to distribute the body's weight, reducing pressure on your bones and joints.

- If done intensively as a vigorous full body cardiovascular workout, it uses 90 per cent of the body's muscles. You can also try it at a more relaxed pace.

- As part of weight control, Nordic walking can burn up to 65 per cent more calories in a session than an average walking pace.

- Being in the great outdoors and breathing fresh air while completing a vigorous workout is a mood booster, and joining Nordic walking groups give an opportunity for companionship and fun.

THE RIGHT POLES FOR YOU

Selecting the right poles and making sure they are the correct height for you is essential. Adjustable poles allow for easier height adjustments, though single-piece poles are more robust and better able to support your weight. Keep your elbows at right angles while holding the poles, and check that they measure 65 per cent of your overall height, excluding the tips. All terrain tips allow you to walk anywhere. Otherwise, you will need to change the tips to suit where you intend to walk: rubber for concrete and hard surfaces, or a pointed tip for grass, beaches, or softer ground.

NORDIC WALKING TECHNIQUE

So, how do you begin? Follow the basic walking technique (see pp62–67), holding good posture with a straight back.

1. Place the pole straps around your wrists, and imagine the poles have become extensions of your arms, noting that the poles will always be slightly behind you.

2. Hold the pole firmly each time it hits the ground. Then, as you move forward and your arm moves back, open your hand to the release position. Grip it again as your arm moves forward to replant, and repeat.

Single arm poling

There are two different techniques that you can try. The first, better for beginners, is to walk naturally with arms in opposition to your feet. As you strike the ground with your right front heel, you also plant your front pole. You can use the same side as your leading foot on the right, or the opposite pole on left, depending on which feels more comfortable. As you move forward, the pole still in the planted position moves behind you, ready to repeat on the opposite side.

Double arm poling

The second way is called "double poling" where you plant both poles symmetrically in front, and then pull yourself forward as you take 2–3 steps, replant your poles, and repeat. This technique can be a lot of fun and works really well if you are moving fast – whether over uneven terrain, going downhill, or just to raise the intensity of your workout. Double poling also offers better stability and balance for anyone moving at a more moderate pace who needs the support.

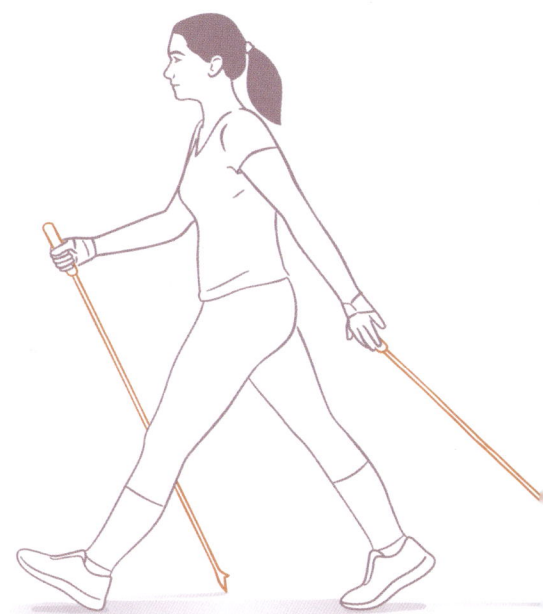

LESSONS AND GROUPS

If you're still not sure, joining a Nordic walking community or club brings together like-minded people socially, where you can share their experience. Or, take a few lessons to learn good basic technique. You can Nordic walk anywhere over any terrain, but the same tips always apply; keep well hydrated and always warm up before and cool down after any workout.

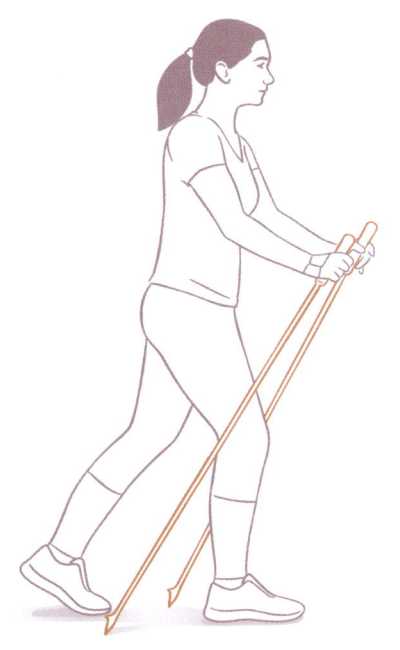

Competitive race walking

If you love walking fast and would like to push yourself that bit further, discover a different type of challenge altogether with either speed or race walking. It is exciting and motivating and no matter how many times you take part in a race, it feels incredible to cross the finish line and receive your medal.

Unless they are specifically for race walkers, most competitive races take place on roads and are primarily for runners. Provided you are able to complete the distance within the official finishing time, these are still ideal for fast walkers to take part in. Some marathons now even offer a walking category. Often a fast walker will match the pace of a runner, so you should not be discouraged from entering. However, it is important to be aware of the event rules and the courtesy required when competing with runners.

Road races are fun events, and many double as money-raising avenues for charity (see pp138–139), although some people will be taking part simply to win or achieve a personal best. There is a multitude of different distances that you an choose from, so you can start with a shorter distance and build up to a marathon or more over time.

ENTERING A MARATHON

A marathon is 42.2km (26¼ miles) long, and can take on average between five and eight hours to complete, which is a significant amount of time to be on your feet. Never underestimate the training needed to ensure you finish a marathon. You should allow yourself a minimum of 12 weeks to prepare, particularly if you are aiming for a good finishing time. If you have never walked before, you may need to allow 12 to 18 weeks to train. Your aim is to reach a fast pace that you can constantly sustain throughout the distance of the challenge. The pace required will be determined either by your personal ambition, or the official times set by the organizers – see the training plan on pp162–167).

Fifty per cent of walking a successful marathon is your mental approach and the self belief that you can achieve your goal. Using visualization to picture yourself with the medal and repeating mantras (see p129) are powerful tools in preparation. You will also need to think carefully about your diet and nutritional needs towards the end of your training. For advice on what you

> "Fifty per cent of walking a successful marathon is your mental approach and the self belief that you can achieve your goal."

need to eat and drink on the days leading up to the marathon, see p117. On the day, follow the number one rule: do not make any changes to your clothing, footwear, or food. Keep everything as you have practised in your training and preparation. Even if you need to tape your feet due to warm weather conditions, try it out before the challenge day so there are no surprises!

SPEED WALKING AND RACEWALKING

Speed walkers using normal technique (see pp62–67) walk at a fast pace to reach a constant 8kph (5mph) or more. At this speed, your body naturally feels that it wants to run. However, if you continue walking, it's at this point that speed walkers will begin using more energy and burn more calories mile for mile than runners. While it is relatively easy to progress from power to speed walking, racewalking is a competitive sport, represented in the Commonwealth and Olympic Games with record walking speeds of 13.6–15kph (8.5–9.3mph). It demands greater endurance, similar to a long distance runner, as well as specific technique and form.

Important rules in racewalking

While the starting posture, arms, and stance are the same as in regular walking (see pp60–61), the difference is the two key rules that must be strictly followed. First, one foot must always have contact with the ground, so the advancing foot must make contact, before the back foot can lift. In competition, having air under both feet as a runner can lead to disqualification. Second, as the lead foot makes contact with the ground, the knee on that leg must be straight. It is the combination of the straight leg, the fast hip rotation as the weight is transferred from side to side, and the shorter stride, that makes it easier and more efficient to achieve a higher stride frequency.

To reach high levels of speed when walking, it is important to take more steps per minute, which can be 180–200pm. While Olympians may be reaching some extraordinary levels, racewalking clubs worldwide welcome and encourage all ages and abilities to start walking distances from 1.6km (1 mile) to 161km (100 miles) or more. Coaching is readily available and as both speed and racewalking are low impact, with a low injury risk, if you're looking for speed, why not give them a go?

BE PREPARED

Having taken part in many marathons, my number one tip is being prepared.

Make sure your clothing, socks, shoes, and even the underwear that you intend to wear for the challenge is all put to the test well in advance. If it works, don't change a thing on the day. Tape your feet in sensitive areas as a preventative measure. Keep to simple energy-giving foods, and stay well hydrated (see p117). Prepare everything you will need the night before, and sleep well ... good luck!

Challenge walking

There has never been an easier time to set yourself a personal goal, by signing up for a challenge. There are so many to choose from, with something for every ability and ambition. A charity challenge also offers the added benefit of raising money and awareness for a good cause. You just need decide when, where, and what goal to set yourself.

FOR FIRST-TIMERS

I know only too well how exciting it is when you have set your mind on signing up for a challenge. Often the eagerness and excitement overrides everything. Before you make any decisions as to whether it is a 5km (3 miles) for a local cause or a long trek, investigate exactly what will be required. In particular, find out if there are time limits on reaching the finish line, or any costs involved. Depending on your level of fitness, which can be easy to overlook in your enthusiasm, are you able to commit to the training needed to achieve your goal?

If you are looking for a less demanding challenge, an ideal distance is 5km (3 miles) or 10km (6 miles). Preparation may take only three to four weeks, while a full marathon, especially if it is an official running event, will require a dedicated training plan of around 12–14 weeks (see pp162–167). Training for events such as long-distance hikes or ultra challenges will follow a similar timeframe (see pp168–179). If you are joining an event, such as the New York City Marathon, you will need a power walking pace of 7–8kph (4.5–5mph) to ensure you finish in time to get that well-deserved medal!

Other events may not be so demanding, and are more accommodating towards mixed abilities and families taking part. Consider whether you would prefer to walk alone, or join a group. The team spirit of walking with others can be a real source of encouragement, and a boost to your motivation when you need it most. It is incredibly sociable, and often the source of many long-lasting friendships.

SPONSORSHIP AND FUNDRAISING

If you are taking part in a challenge for a cause, there can be high level demand for charity places to enter some events, outweighing the availability. Often these come with a requirement to raise a specified minimum amount of sponsorship. Before signing up, think about whether or not you will be able to raise the funds required, as in some cases it can be quite high. Your chosen charity will help you with plenty of inspirational ideas on how to fundraise. However, be aware that not meeting the expected level of funds could mean the charity loses money.

THERE'S ALWAYS ANOTHER LEVEL!

Your first challenge experience will hopefully inspire you to take part in more. There are always new challenges, distances, and terrains to discover. Any that involve travelling to another country add another level of excitement to your adventure. Some charities offer reimbursement of travelling costs, in exchange for raising sponsorship. The result is a great exchange: you get to travel, and the charity receives much-needed funds.

Walk the Walk, the charity I founded, specializes in organizing walking challenges around the world, while raising money for vital cancer causes, and cancer prevention. Most well-known are our flagship and iconic MoonWalk events, the original and first challenge of its kind, where people complete a marathon overnight. Held in London, Scotland, and Iceland it attracts every age and every ability to take part. We also offer a wide range of walks and treks. Some of my favourites are the New York City Marathon – an amazing experience; The Nijmegen Marches – 4 days of trekking in the Netherlands; and our Camino challenges – ancient routes with a modern twist. Perhaps today is the day to sign up for your first walking challenge!

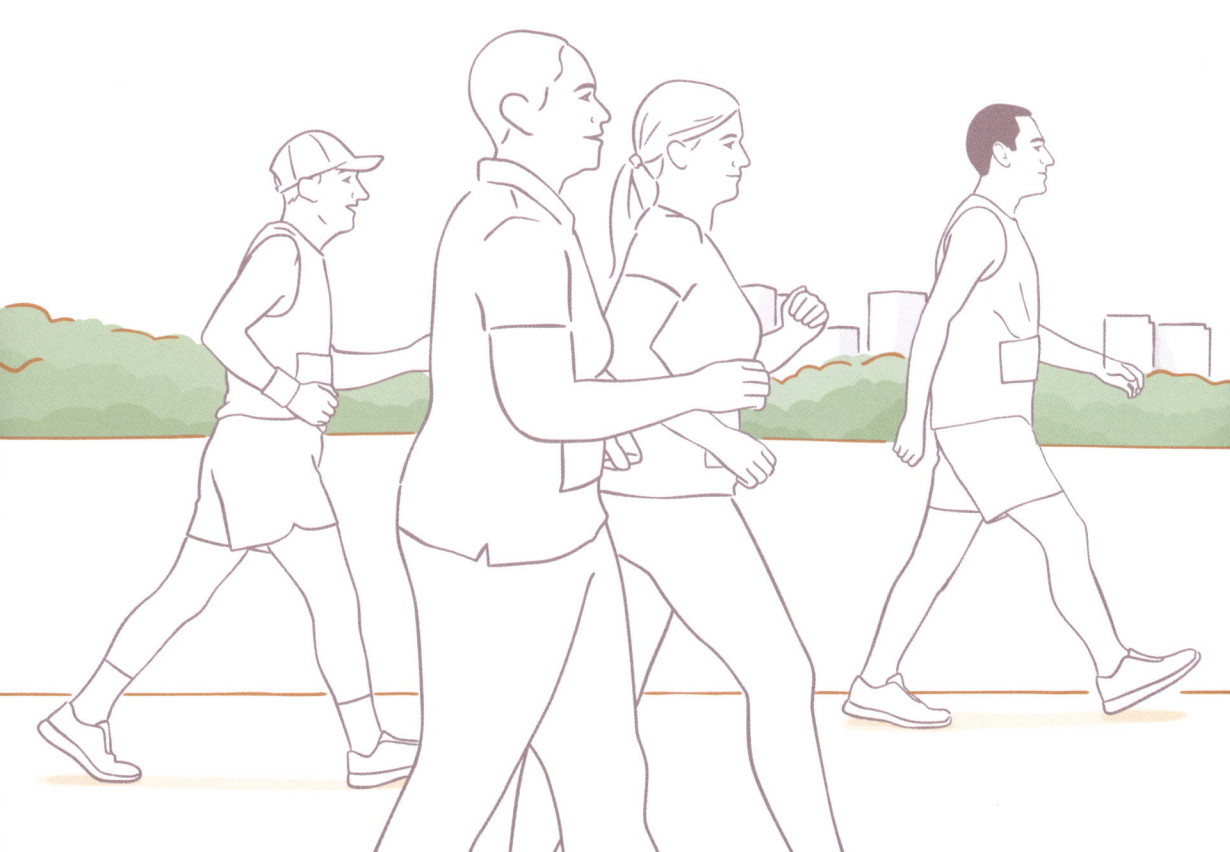

Healthy walking

Everywhere you turn, you'll find a wealth of information highlighting the health benefits of walking. But how do we know what constitutes a healthy amount? How far and for how long should we walk? Is it more important to focus on the distance or the time spent walking? Perhaps your goal is simply to use walking as a way to feel fitter and healthier.

Well, there is good news! Researchers from Cambridge University have carried out one of the largest studies to date, covering more than 30 million participants from 94 large study cohorts. According to the research, just 11 minutes a day (75 minutes a week) of moderately intense physical activity, such as a brisk walk, can make a difference to your overall mental and physical fitness. It could also lower the risk of heart disease, cancer, and other critical conditions.

LESSEN SICK DAYS AND CRAVINGS

A Harvard study found that people who walked for a minimum of 20 minutes a day for five days of the week had 43 per cent fewer sick days than those who only exercised once a week or less. When you do find yourself in stressful situations, a 15-minute brisk walk can also reduce cravings for chocolate or alcohol usually associated with stress. In short, these studies show that doing some physical activity is certainly better than none. Just a few minutes a day can make a significant impact on your overall health.

BUILDING WALKING INTO YOUR LIFE

There are plenty of very compelling arguments throughout this book as to why you should incorporate walking into your life. While 11 minutes doesn't seem much, making the leap from thinking about it to actually doing it can be a challenge. Start with five-minute segments, which you could spread across the whole day. Or, if you have a smart watch, track your steps from the moment you get up in the morning to going to bed at night. The aim is to capture every step and walk a minimum of about 5,000 steps (3.2km/2 miles) over the entire day. This can be quite an eye opener; you may suddenly discover that you are actually doing more than you thought. Or, you might be horrified at how little you are doing.

Find opportunities to walk
Get creative by finding short time slots within your day to move; if you can do it outside in the fresh air, all the better (see p24). A short walk after a meal helps with digestion. It releases oxygen throughout the body, increases levels of endorphins to boost your spirits, and makes you feel more energized. There is nothing like a walk to solve a problem. When possible, use stairs instead of lifts, and walk up escalators rather than letting them do all the work. Try a walking and talking meeting, or pace the room when you are on the phone – it all counts.

IMPORTANCE OF FREQUENCY

Just by making these simple changes to your day, you will find that your sleep improves, allowing you to wake up feeling more energetic (see p25). As with any activity, consistency is key, so try to walk 3.2km (2 miles) on as many days of the week as possible. Your pace and intensity are not important – these will both build quite naturally – and you could very soon be walking 30 minutes each day.

"A short walk releases oxygen throughout the body, increases levels of endorphins to boost your spirits, and makes you feel more energized."

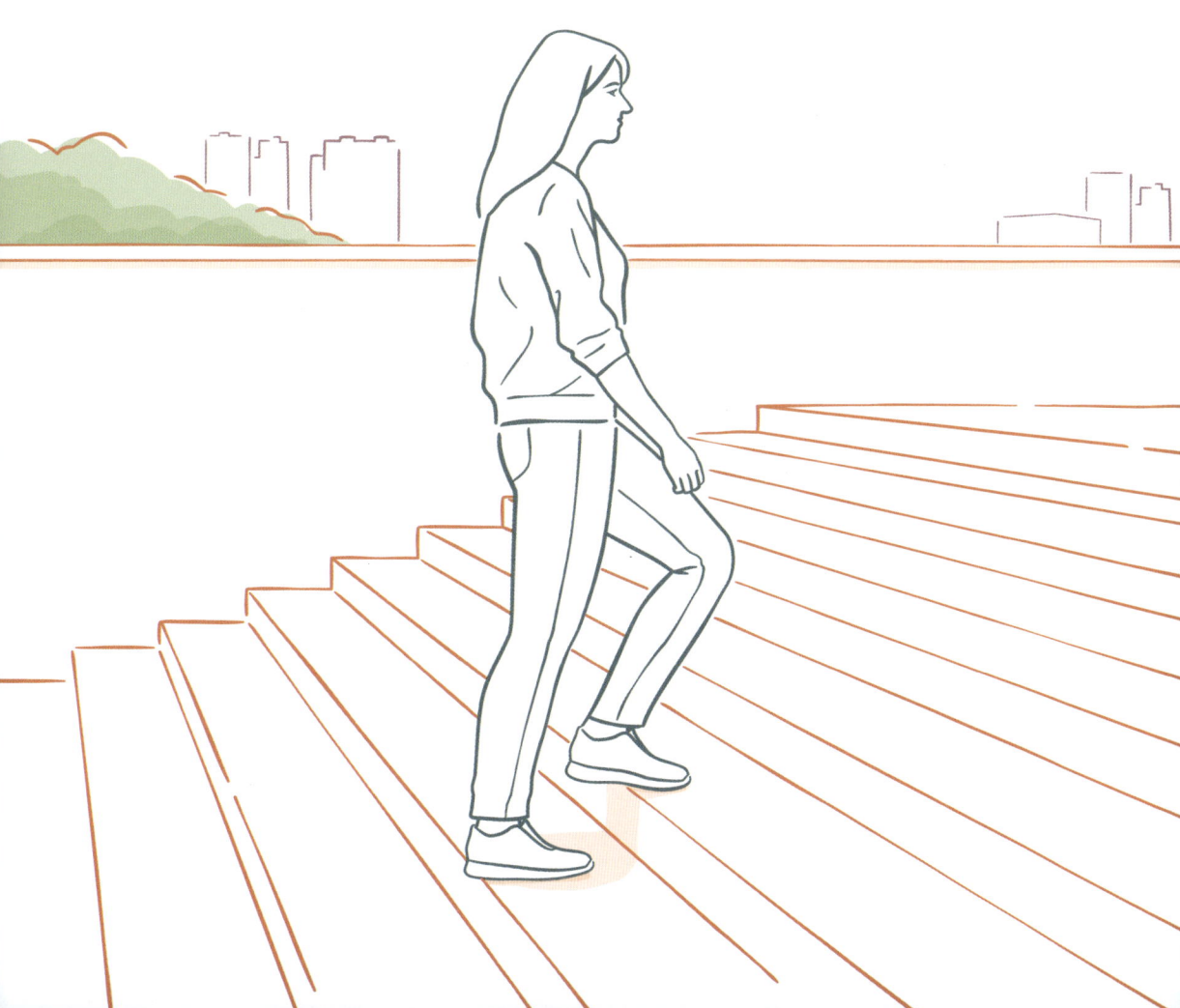

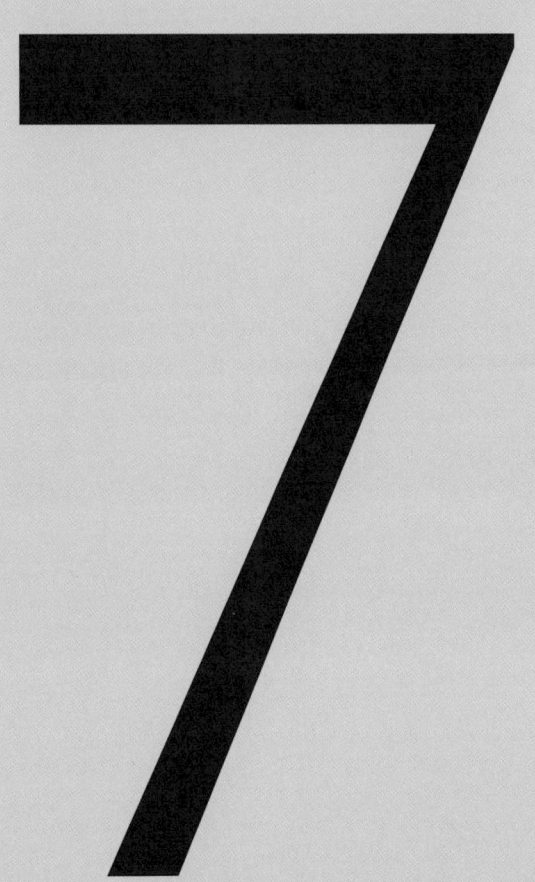

Training programmes

Making a commitment to a training programme can feel overwhelming, but I hope you will also feel excited. The rewards and satisfaction of sticking to an exercise regime come not just from reaching a goal, but from discovering new strengths and abilities within yourself, and enjoying the achievements that you have gained on the way.

A daily walk

LEVEL: 1 / TOTAL: 12 WEEKS

This programme aims to help you reach a fitness level where you can walk for one hour a day. Before you begin, you must be able to walk continuously for 15 minutes at any pace. If this feels uncomfortable, try tracking and then increasing your AM–PM steps until you feel ready to begin.

WEEKS 1–6

Week 1
Begin by allowing your body to adapt to the idea of walking every day. Notice how you feel and congratulate yourself on taking the first step. Your pace is not important – just enjoy the time you are creating for yourself.

Week 2
If you don't feel ready to move on, repeat Week 1. If you are ready, then in your second week, you will repeat the time you are walking, but you may find you walk further in the same time. Wearing a smart watch is a reliable way to track your steps, pace, and time. It is also useful to use the heart-rate monitor to check on your exertion. You should be able to talk as you walk!

Weeks 3–4
By now you should begin to feel more energized. If you are comfortable with the length of time you are walking, try walking further within the same time period. Also track your AM–PM steps. You are now walking every day – what an achievement!

Weeks 5–6
From Week 5 the walking time begins to increase, as well as your pace. Apart from having favourite walks, make sure that you continually plot new ones to keep yourself motivated. As you progress, you will continue to walk further within the same time period.

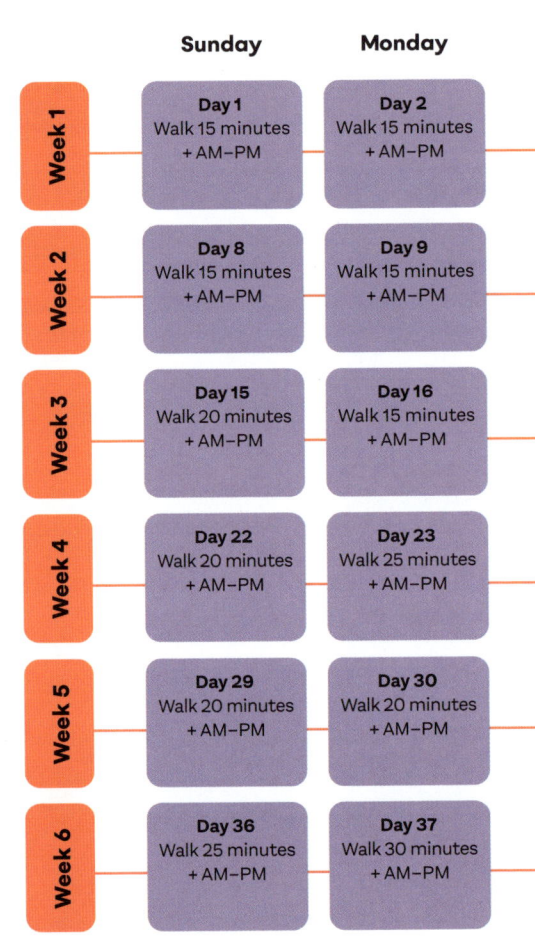

Other pages to help you: Using a smartphone and apps, see p52 • Using a heart-rate monitor, see p53 • Walking technique, see pp62–67 • Posture, see pp60–61 • Breathing, see pp98–101 • Fit walking into your day, see pp12–13 • Warming up and cooling down, see pp90–91; Warm-up and cool-down routines, see p94 • Stretch and strengthen routine, see p95

Key — Walk days | MPW: Minutes per week

AM–PM refers to tracking your steps from the moment you get up to bedtime, with the aim of covering 3.2km (2 miles) throughout the day.

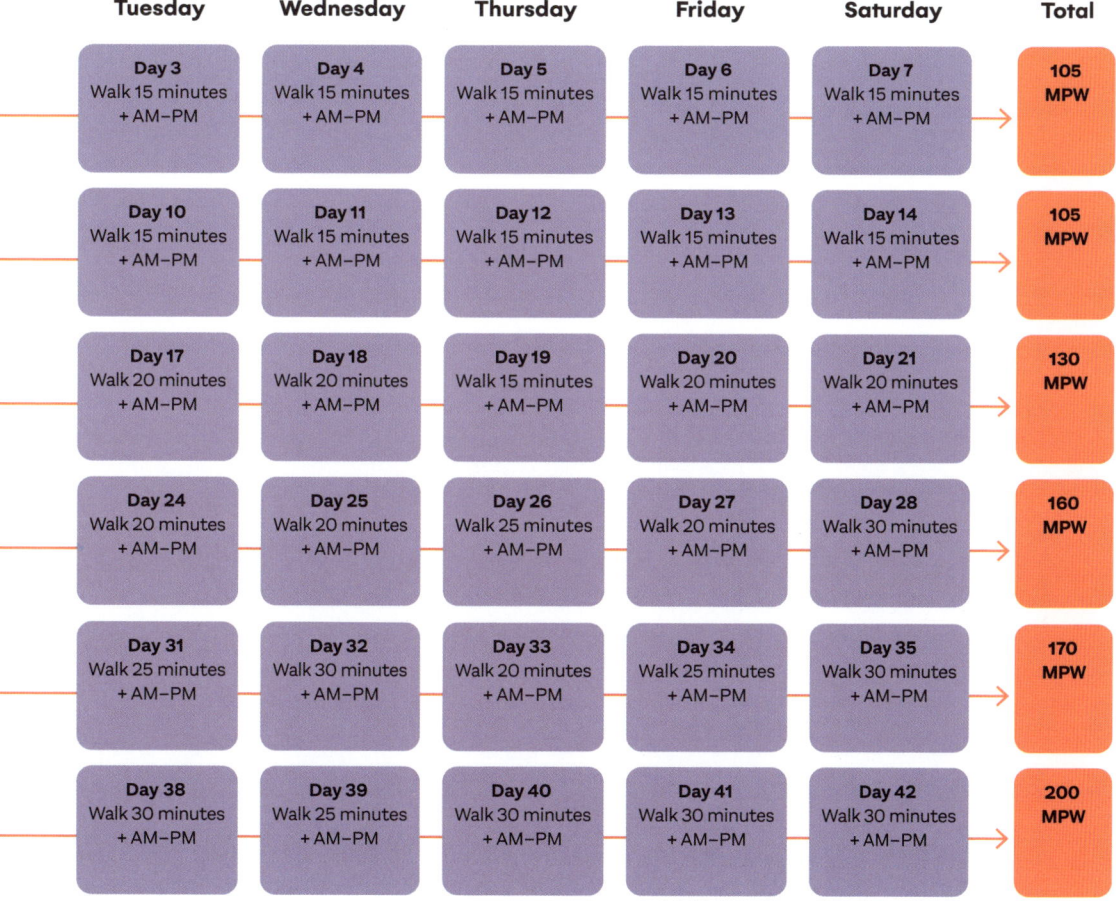

TRAINING PROGRAMMES 145

A DAILY WALK WEEKS 7–12

Weeks 7–8
By now you should be feeling confident with completing a daily walk. Begin working on your technique as this is key to increasing your speed. Make sure you have good posture with your shoulders relaxed and back. Engage your core, tipping your pelvis slightly forward. Even if you have not yet reached a speed where you are using your arms to propel you forward, it is useful to hold them in the right position, right angles at your sides, for when you do want to speed up.

Weeks 9–12
It is a great feeling to experience yourself getting fitter and stronger. With the right technique, walking can achieve a total body workout like nothing else. In these last weeks of the training plan you should be feeling much more confident in your walking ability as you reach your goal of a daily hour of walking.

There is no reason that you should stop when you reach Week 12. However, you may want to set yourself a new goal or challenge. Or, you can continue with your daily hour looking at creative ways to keep your walking fresh. Find new routes and terrains, new speed challenges, walking meditations, and even forming a group to walk with friends. Nordic walking (see pp134–135) is also a fun workout for short distance walkers, presenting a different type of experience, particularly if you go off road. Join a class and not only will you have walking companions, but you will also probably find the instructor will provide the poles. As you count your AM–PM steps, set yourself a weekly challenge of how you can increase your total each week.

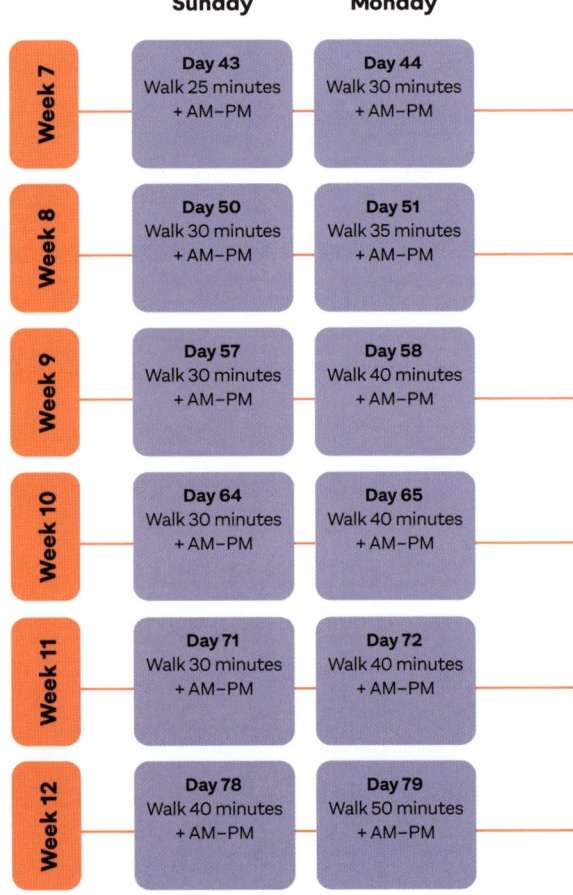

	Sunday	Monday
Week 7	Day 43 Walk 25 minutes + AM–PM	Day 44 Walk 30 minutes + AM–PM
Week 8	Day 50 Walk 30 minutes + AM–PM	Day 51 Walk 35 minutes + AM–PM
Week 9	Day 57 Walk 30 minutes + AM–PM	Day 58 Walk 40 minutes + AM–PM
Week 10	Day 64 Walk 30 minutes + AM–PM	Day 65 Walk 40 minutes + AM–PM
Week 11	Day 71 Walk 30 minutes + AM–PM	Day 72 Walk 40 minutes + AM–PM
Week 12	Day 78 Walk 40 minutes + AM–PM	Day 79 Walk 50 minutes + AM–PM

Other pages to help you: Using a smartphone and apps, see p52 • Using a heart-rate monitor, see p53 • Walking technique, see pp62–67 • Posture, see pp60–61 • Breathing, see pp98–101 • Fit walking into your day, see pp12–13 • Warming up and cooling down, see pp90–91; Warm-up and cool-down routines, see p94 • Stretch and strengthen routine, see p95

Key ■ Walk days | MPW: Minutes per week

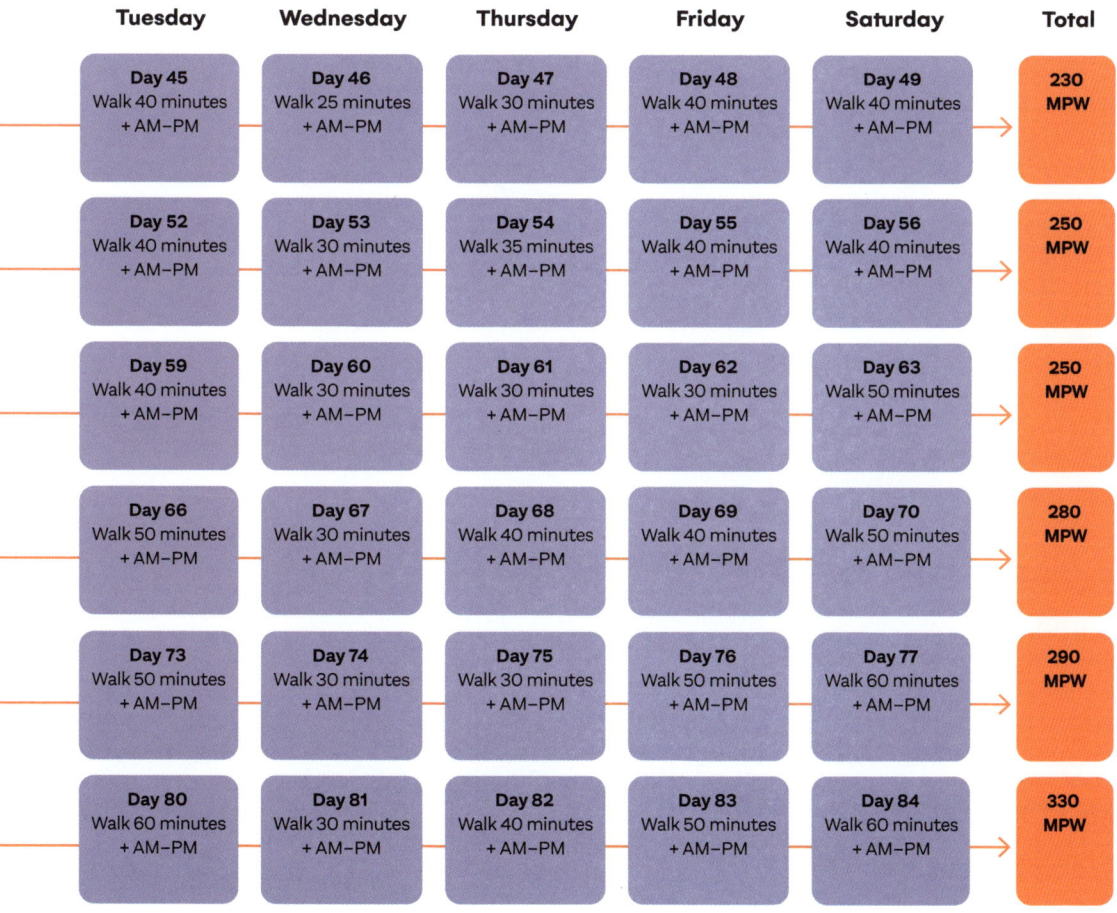

Walking yourself well

LEVEL: 1 / TOTAL: 12 WEEKS

This programme is for anyone who has decided to include walking with purpose into their daily life, or has not been active for a long time and is starting from scratch. The goal is to reach a daily distance of up to 6.43km (4 miles) at a walking pace of 15–18 minutes per 1.6km (1 mile).

WEEKS 1–6

Week 1
Walk 0.8–1.6km (½–1 mile) to determine which distance is the best starting point for you. Walking at a steady pace to suit you means you can focus on achieving the distance.
If you are at all active in your daily life, you may have more stamina than you think. It is more important to get used to the routine of daily walking, but no matter how slow you walk, try to keep a steady and continuous pace.

Week 2
Start getting used to a daily stretch of 5–10 minutes. It will make a big difference to your flexibility. To warm up, stretch for 5 minutes after the first 5 minutes of your walk. To cool down, slow your pace about 10 minutes from the end of your walk, then stretch immediately. Begin to become more aware of how your body feels as you walk, especially your posture.

Weeks 3–4
Introduce other activities into your week. It can be anything you enjoy, such as swimming or dancing.

Weeks 5–6
You are walking further and more often, so begin to add variety to your daily walk by planning different routes.

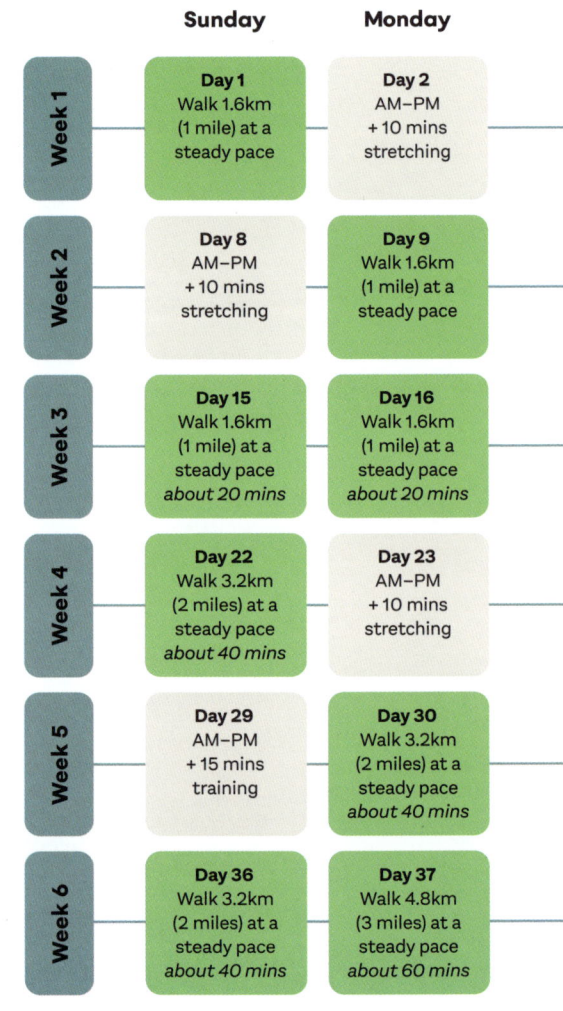

	Sunday	Monday
Week 1	**Day 1** Walk 1.6km (1 mile) at a steady pace	**Day 2** AM–PM +10 mins stretching
Week 2	**Day 8** AM–PM +10 mins stretching	**Day 9** Walk 1.6km (1 mile) at a steady pace
Week 3	**Day 15** Walk 1.6km (1 mile) at a steady pace *about 20 mins*	**Day 16** Walk 1.6km (1 mile) at a steady pace *about 20 mins*
Week 4	**Day 22** Walk 3.2km (2 miles) at a steady pace *about 40 mins*	**Day 23** AM–PM +10 mins stretching
Week 5	**Day 29** AM–PM +15 mins training	**Day 30** Walk 3.2km (2 miles) at a steady pace *about 40 mins*
Week 6	**Day 36** Walk 3.2km (2 miles) at a steady pace *about 40 mins*	**Day 37** Walk 4.8km (3 miles) at a steady pace *about 60 mins*

Before extending the distance, use weeks 1–6 to focus on developing a daily routine. You will find that you will naturally speed up in weeks 7–12. This plan is a guide; try to walk and stretch daily, but most importantly be aware that it has to fit into your life.

Other pages to help you: Any other activity, see pp180–181 • Stretching exercises, see pp84–89 • Warming up and cooling down, see pp90–93

AM–PM refers to tracking your steps from the moment you get up to bedtime, with the aim of covering 3.2km (2 miles) throughout the day.

Key ■ Walk days   ■ AM–PM   ■ Other activity days

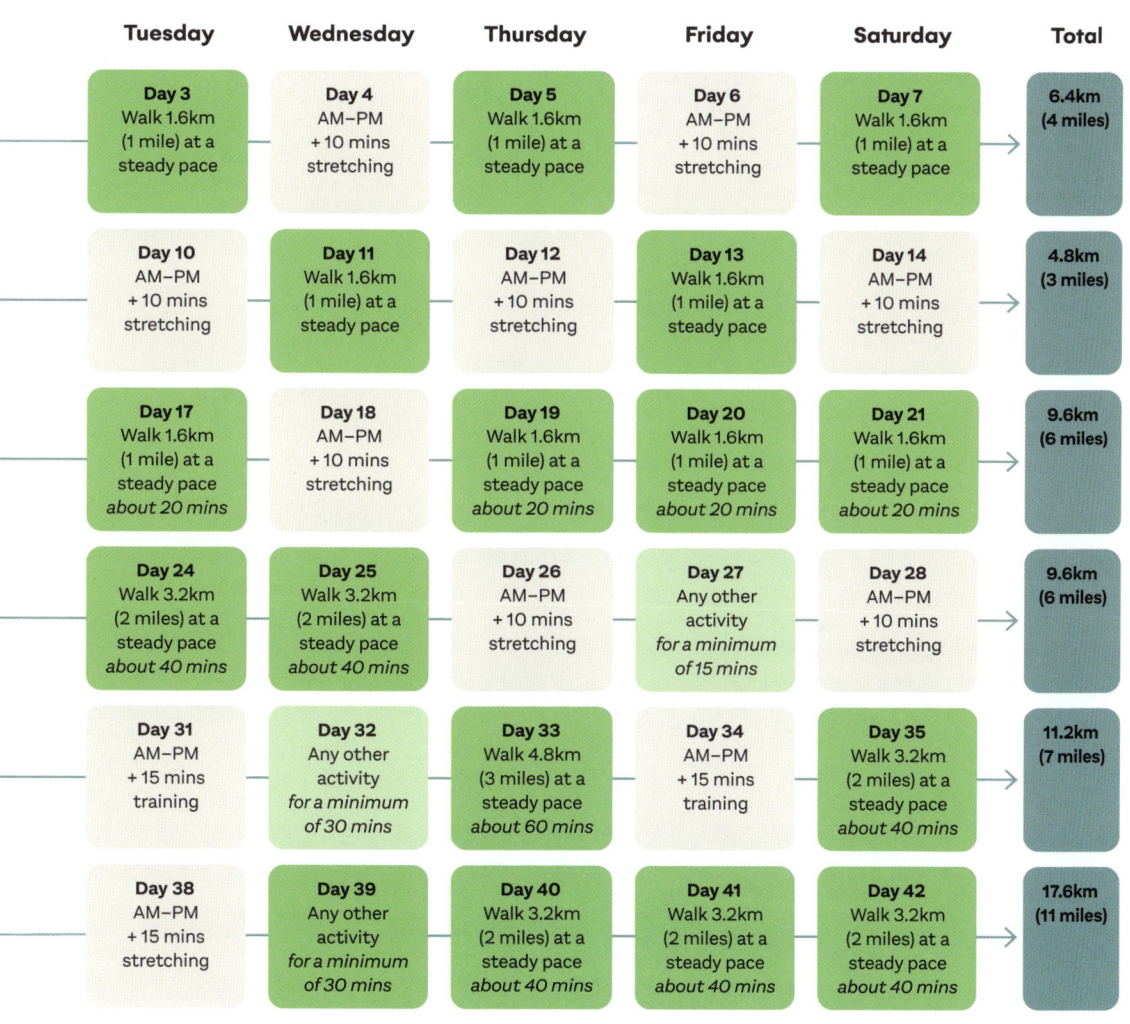

WALKING YOURSELF WELL WEEKS 7–12

Weeks 7–8
You are now walking faster and with purpose, while developing strength and technique. You should feel that you are exerting yourself, but still be able to talk as you walk. If you don't feel ready, go back to Week 5 and complete the last two weeks again. If you feel fine, continue into Weeks 7 and 8.

Track your AM–PM daily steps, including them into every day of your plan. The quality of your steps is more important than the quantity. The faster you move, the more it will benefit you.

Weeks 9–12
Listen to your body, and if you find the pace too hard, take a few steps back.

By Week 12 you should feel stronger, fitter, and confidently able to walk 6.4kph (4mph) as well as achieving your AM–PM goal. Congratulations!

When you have completed this programme, you may wish to try the short-distance programme (see pp144–147).

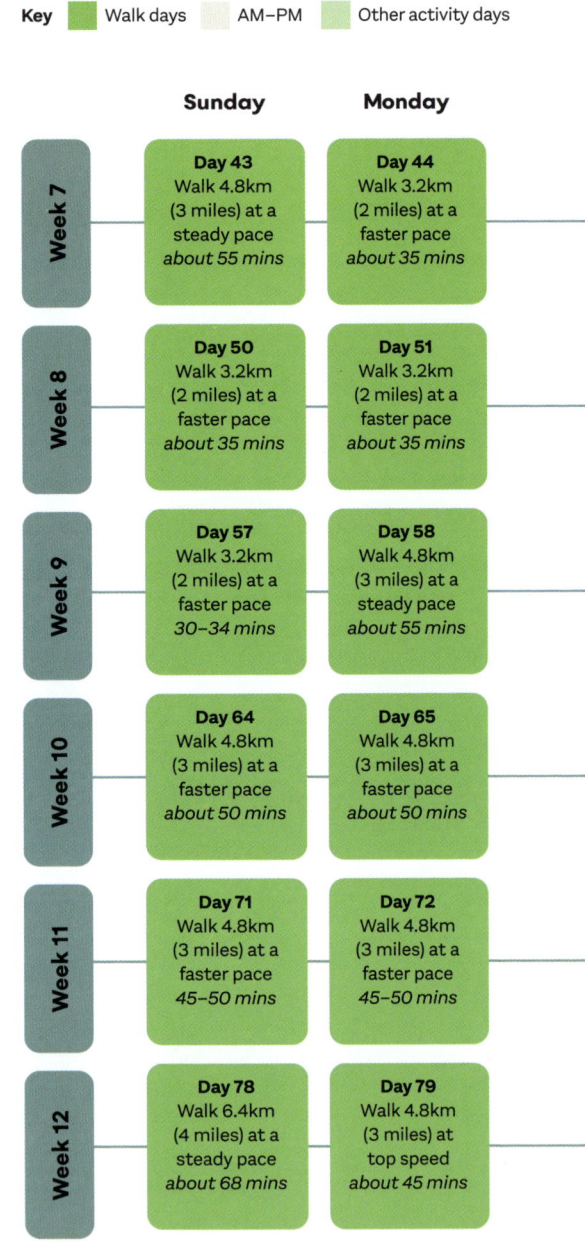

150   WALK YOURSELF WELL

Other pages to help you: Any other activity, see pp180–181 • Stretching exercises, see pp84–89 • Warming up and cooling down, see pp90–93

Tuesday	Wednesday	Thursday	Friday	Saturday	Total
Day 45 Any other activity *for a minimum of 30 mins*	**Day 46** AM–PM + 15 mins stretching	**Day 47** Walk 4.8km (3 miles) at a steady pace *about 55 mins*	**Day 48** Walk 3.2km (2 miles) at a faster pace *about 35 mins*	**Day 49** Walk 1.6km (1 mile) at top speed *about 18 mins*	**17.6km (11 miles)**
Day 52 Walk 3.2km (2 miles) at a faster pace *about 32 mins*	**Day 53** Walk 4.8km (3 miles) at a steady pace *about 50 mins*	**Day 54** Any other activity *for a minimum of 15 mins*	**Day 55** AM–PM + 15 mins stretching	**Day 56** Walk 3.2km (2 miles) at a faster pace *about 32 mins*	**17.6km (11 miles)**
Day 59 Any other activity *for a minimum of 30 mins*	**Day 60** Walk 3.2km (2 miles) at a faster pace *30–34 mins*	**Day 61** Walk 4.8km (3 miles) at a faster pace *about 48 mins*	**Day 62** AM–PM + 15 mins stretching	**Day 63** Walk 3.2km (2 miles) at a faster pace *30–34 mins*	**19.2km (12 miles)**
Day 66 AM–PM + 15 mins stretching	**Day 67** Any other activity *for a minimum of 30 mins*	**Day 68** Walk 3.2km (2 miles) *about 30 mins*	**Day 69** Walk 4.8km (3 miles) at a faster pace *about 50 mins*	**Day 70** Walk 4.8km (3 miles) at a faster pace *about 50 mins*	**22.4km (14 miles)**
Day 73 AM–PM + 15 mins stretching	**Day 74** Any other activity *for a minimum of 30 mins*	**Day 75** Walk 4.8km (3 miles) at a faster pace *about 45–50 mins*	**Day 76** Walk 4.8km (3 miles) at a faster pace *about 45–50 mins*	**Day 77** Walk 4.8km (3 miles) at a faster pace *about 45–50 mins*	**24km (15 miles)**
Day 80 Any other activity *for a minimum of 30 mins*	**Day 81** Walk 6.4km (4 miles) at a steady pace *about 70–98 mins*	**Day 82** Walk 4.8km (3 miles) at top speed *about 45–50 mins*	**Day 83** AM–PM + 15 mins stretching	**Day 84** Walk 6.4km (4 miles) at top speed *about 60 mins*	**28.8km (18 miles)**

TRAINING PROGRAMMES

Weight control and fitness

LEVEL: 2 / TOTAL: 12 WEEKS

To control weight and increase your fitness, you will need to walk continuously for a minimum of 45 minutes, four times a week. The amount of calories you burn will depend on various factors, including how fast you walk. Your aim is 1.6km (1 mile) in 15–17 minutes.

WEEKS 1–6

Walking will help you to control your weight, tone muscle, and increase your overall fitness. However, the results will depend on your age, weight, and your starting point, combined with eating a healthy diet to ensure long-lasting results. There are aids such as using a smart watch to monitor your body's vital signs; specifically heart rate and movement. Apps are also available for your phone on which you can track your calories, record weight, and check blood pressure. There are also scales available that will record your body fat. If you are not used to any physical activity and unsure of your health and ability, seek medical advice before starting this programme.

Weeks 1–6
Beginning to walk at a steady pace means that you could be walking more energetically than usual. You should start by aiming to walk for 20 minutes per 1.6km (1 mile). It's important to feel an increase in your heart rate, but you should still be able to hold a conversation while walking. If you're finding the distance challenging, try walking with the support of Nordic poles. Although you will probably move faster using the poles, the effort will seem easier, and this could be just the motivation that works for you in the first few weeks of your training. Make time for stretching, both before and after your walk.

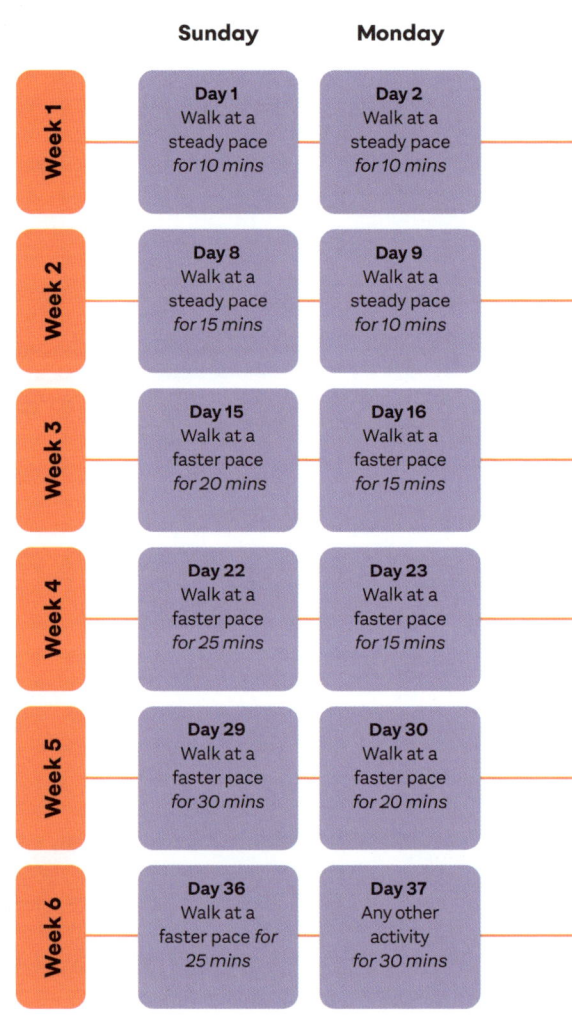

	Sunday	Monday
Week 1	Day 1 Walk at a steady pace *for 10 mins*	Day 2 Walk at a steady pace *for 10 mins*
Week 2	Day 8 Walk at a steady pace *for 15 mins*	Day 9 Walk at a steady pace *for 10 mins*
Week 3	Day 15 Walk at a faster pace *for 20 mins*	Day 16 Walk at a faster pace *for 15 mins*
Week 4	Day 22 Walk at a faster pace *for 25 mins*	Day 23 Walk at a faster pace *for 15 mins*
Week 5	Day 29 Walk at a faster pace *for 30 mins*	Day 30 Walk at a faster pace *for 20 mins*
Week 6	Day 36 Walk at a faster pace *for 25 mins*	Day 37 Any other activity *for 30 mins*

Use this programme as a guide, adapting it to fit your life. Your ultimate goal is to achieve a good pace and to maintain it for an hour. As you progress, you will find that you are able to walk further in the same amount of time. Start at a pace that is a little faster than your normal pace and increase distance and speed only when you are ready.

Other pages to help you: Walking for weight control pp16–17 • Using a smartphone and apps, see p52 • Walking technique, see pp62–67 • Nordic walking, see pp134–135 • Foods for health and fitness, see pp116–119 • Warming up and cooling down, see pp90–93 • Stretch and strengthen routine, see p95 • Treadmill walking, see pp124–125

Key — Walk days | MPW: Minutes per week

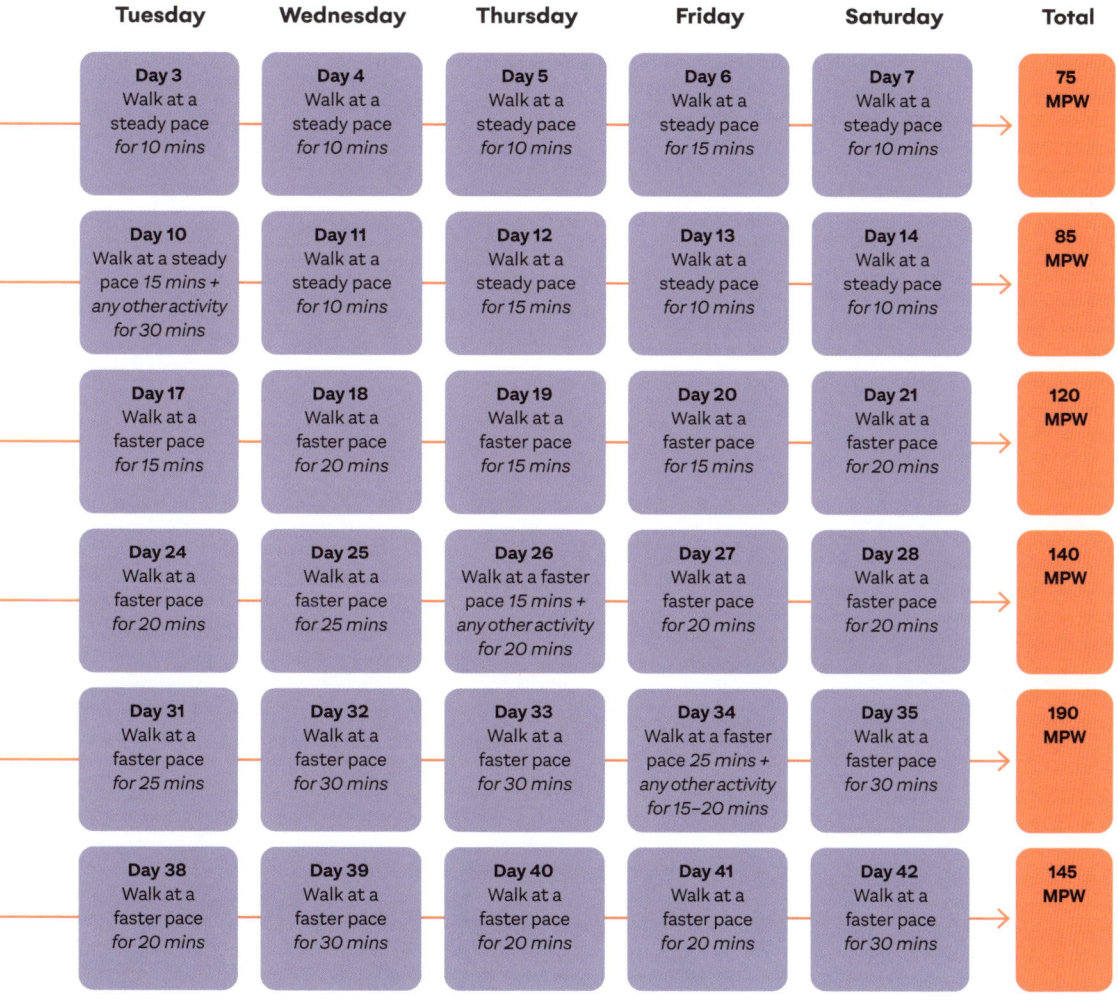

	Tuesday	Wednesday	Thursday	Friday	Saturday	Total
	Day 3 Walk at a steady pace *for 10 mins*	**Day 4** Walk at a steady pace *for 10 mins*	**Day 5** Walk at a steady pace *for 10 mins*	**Day 6** Walk at a steady pace *for 15 mins*	**Day 7** Walk at a steady pace *for 10 mins*	**75 MPW**
	Day 10 Walk at a steady pace *15 mins + any other activity for 30 mins*	**Day 11** Walk at a steady pace *for 10 mins*	**Day 12** Walk at a steady pace *for 15 mins*	**Day 13** Walk at a steady pace *for 10 mins*	**Day 14** Walk at a steady pace *for 10 mins*	**85 MPW**
	Day 17 Walk at a faster pace *for 15 mins*	**Day 18** Walk at a faster pace *for 20 mins*	**Day 19** Walk at a faster pace *for 15 mins*	**Day 20** Walk at a faster pace *for 15 mins*	**Day 21** Walk at a faster pace *for 20 mins*	**120 MPW**
	Day 24 Walk at a faster pace *for 20 mins*	**Day 25** Walk at a faster pace *for 25 mins*	**Day 26** Walk at a faster pace *15 mins + any other activity for 20 mins*	**Day 27** Walk at a faster pace *for 20 mins*	**Day 28** Walk at a faster pace *for 20 mins*	**140 MPW**
	Day 31 Walk at a faster pace *for 25 mins*	**Day 32** Walk at a faster pace *for 30 mins*	**Day 33** Walk at a faster pace *for 30 mins*	**Day 34** Walk at a faster pace *25 mins + any other activity for 15–20 mins*	**Day 35** Walk at a faster pace *for 30 mins*	**190 MPW**
	Day 38 Walk at a faster pace *for 20 mins*	**Day 39** Walk at a faster pace *for 30 mins*	**Day 40** Walk at a faster pace *for 20 mins*	**Day 41** Walk at a faster pace *for 20 mins*	**Day 42** Walk at a faster pace *for 30 mins*	**145 MPW**

TRAINING PROGRAMMES

WEIGHT CONTROL AND FITNESS WEEKS 7–12

Weeks 7–8
By now you'll have a routine in place and be developing a variety of favourite walks. You should also be able to walk further in the same amount of time. Now is a good time to introduce a different activity to your training plan. This must be something that you enjoy, is readily accessible, and will also increase your heart rate, such as swimming, dancing, or using kettlebell weights. You also have the option to include hill walking in these weeks. Hill walking will make your body work harder and burn more calories. If you are not yet ready for this, include it at a later time.

Weeks 9–12
These final weeks of the training plan are all about speed. By now you should be able to reach a 14–16 minute pace per 1.6km (1 mile). Try challenging yourself to cover different terrain, collating a variety of walks that will keep you engaged and motivated. Reaching 12 weeks is a great achievement, so well done to you. For weight management you can continue the plan, by increasing the distance and speed that you walk within the set time, or increase the time as well. This is an effective way to increase your fitness. Or, you could feel you are ready to take on a challenge. Whatever you choose, by continuing to walk and by making healthier choices, there is every chance that you can maintain your ideal weight.

Dont forget to include your daily AM–PM step count on top of your timed distance. Put together, it all adds up!

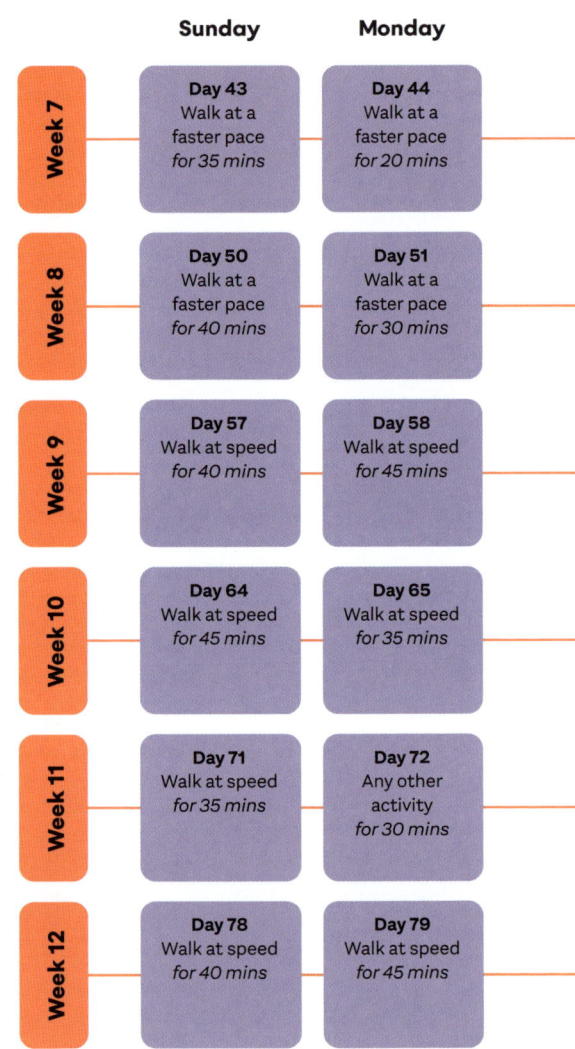

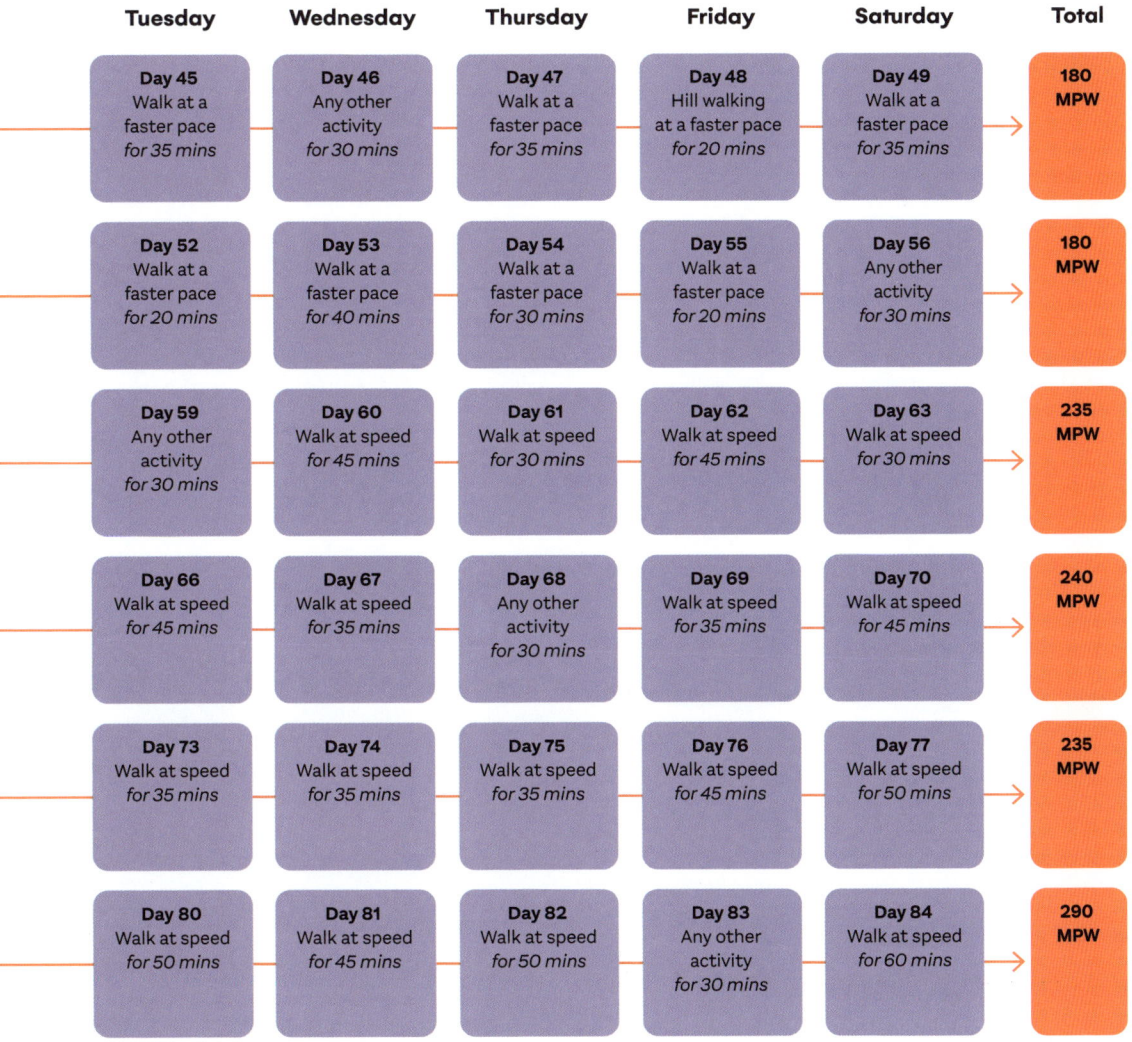

Intermediate: muscle strength and stamina

LEVEL: 3 / TOTAL: 12 WEEKS

If you are able to walk 6.4km (4 miles) at a constant pace, and keen to build your strength and stamina, you are ready for this level. The intermediate training plan not only includes daily stretching and strengthening, it will help to increase your fitness, tone your body, and develop your technique and walking speed.

WEEKS 1–4

Weeks 1–2
The aim of this plan is focused on being active every day in some way. The combination of walking faster and further, regular stretching and strengthening, as well as enjoying other activities, will develop your core strength and stamina. You will also be building greater flexibility, which will increase your range of movement. In addition, you'll be helping to relieve tight muscles in your ankles, shins, and hips, which is very common when starting to walk at speed over longer distances.

As for other activities, try something that either you know you will enjoy, or something you have always wanted to have a go at. Including sports such as swimming, kettlebells, or Pilates, is a good way to cross train, as well as adding variety to your active week.

Weeks 3–4
Hill walking begins in Week 3. Look for new routes with hills, or use a treadmill. If the latter, be creative with the variety of programmes you set. One of the many benefits of including inclines is how fast it can increase your walking strength. Core stability sessions are also

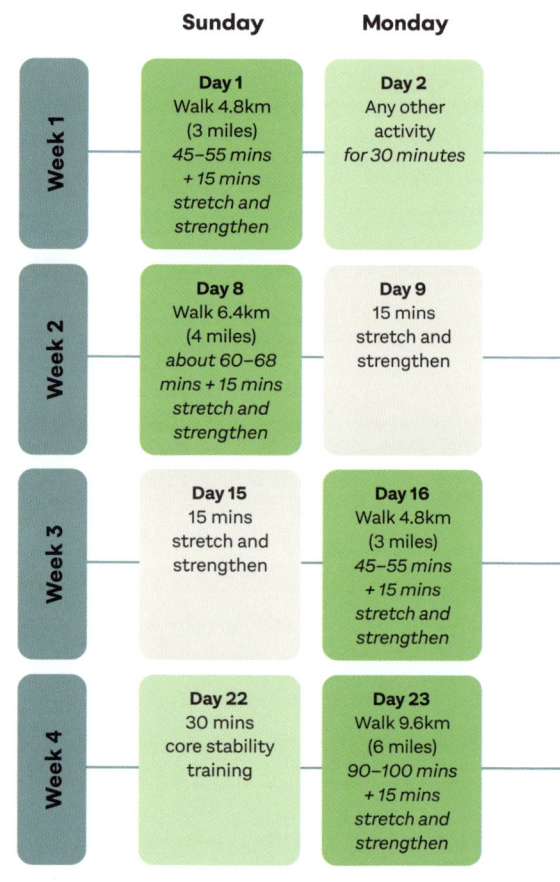

	Sunday	Monday
Week 1	**Day 1** Walk 4.8km (3 miles) 45–55 mins + 15 mins stretch and strengthen	**Day 2** Any other activity for 30 minutes
Week 2	**Day 8** Walk 6.4km (4 miles) about 60–68 mins + 15 mins stretch and strengthen	**Day 9** 15 mins stretch and strengthen
Week 3	**Day 15** 15 mins stretch and strengthen	**Day 16** Walk 4.8km (3 miles) 45–55 mins + 15 mins stretch and strengthen
Week 4	**Day 22** 30 mins core stability training	**Day 23** Walk 9.6km (6 miles) 90–100 mins + 15 mins stretch and strengthen

included in Week 4. Try Pilates, or swing a kettlebell; both are really good core workouts that you can do at home, or in a gym. Using this programme, form a regular workout plan that fits into your life. To begin, work on stamina and speed separately. You will find that over the weeks they do eventually come together. Use the times given here as approximate goals for which you should aim. Always follow a hard training day with an easier one.

Other pages to help you: Using a smartphone and apps, see p52 • Treadmill walking, see pp124–125 • Nordic walking, see pp134–135 • Rucking, see pp130–131 • Upper and lower body stretches, see pp84–87 • Before and after walking, see pp90–93 • Leg stretches, pp78–79

Key — Walk days — Stretch and strengthen — Other activity days

Tuesday	Wednesday	Thursday	Friday	Saturday	Total
Day 3 15 mins stretch and strengthen	**Day 4** Walk 4.8km (3 miles) 45–55 mins + 15 mins stretch and strengthen	**Day 5** 15 mins stretch and strengthen	**Day 6** Walk 4.8km (3 miles) 45–55 mins + 15 mins stretch and strengthen	**Day 7** 15 mins stretch and strengthen	**14.4km (9 miles)**
Day 10 Walk 4.8km (3 miles) 45–55 mins + 15 mins stretch and strengthen	**Day 11** 15 mins stretch and strengthen	**Day 12** Any other activity *for a minimum of 15 minutes*	**Day 13** 15 mins stretch and strengthen	**Day 14** Walk 6.4km (4 miles) 60–68 mins + 15 mins stretch and strengthen	**17.6km (11 miles)**
Day 17 Hill walking 4.8km (3 miles) 50–55 mins + 15 mins stretch and strengthen	**Day 18** 15 mins stretch and strengthen	**Day 19** Any other activity *for a minimum of 30 minutes*	**Day 20** Walk 8km (5 miles) 75–80 mins + 15 mins stretch and strengthen	**Day 21** 15 mins stretch and strengthen	**17.6km (11 miles)**
Day 24 15 mins stretch and strengthen	**Day 25** Walk 8km (5 miles) 75–80 mins + 15 mins stretch and strengthen	**Day 26** 15 mins stretch and strengthen	**Day 27** Walk 4.8km (3 miles) 45–50 mins + 15 mins stretch and strengthen	**Day 28** Any other activity *for a minimum of 30 minutes*	**22.4km (14 miles)**

INTERMEDIATE WEEKS 5-8

Weeks 5-8
By Week 5 you should be feeling stronger and have more energy. You will find that your speed will continue to develop over the next few weeks, particularly if you are also focusing on improving your technique.

Achieving a good heel strike and push off while also keeping your arms at right angles and pumping them no higher than your shoulders can all feel like hard work, but it is worth persevering. It is almost impossible to increase your speed beyond 6.5–7kph (4–4.5mph) without developing good arm technique.

Wearing a smart watch or using your smartphone is a great way of keeping a daily log. The greater the challenge, the more you will appreciate tracking your progress as stepping stones to your ultimate goal.

If you have not tried swinging a kettlebell yet, book into a class to learn the basic movements.

"The greater the challenge, the more you will appreciate tracking your progress as stepping stones to your ultimate goal."

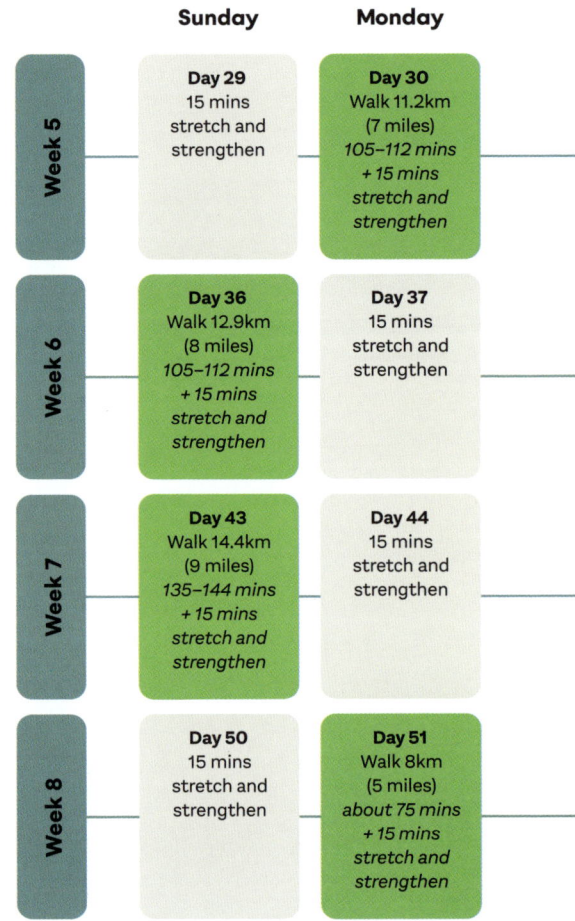

	Sunday	Monday
Week 5	Day 29 15 mins stretch and strengthen	Day 30 Walk 11.2km (7 miles) 105–112 mins + 15 mins stretch and strengthen
Week 6	Day 36 Walk 12.9km (8 miles) 105–112 mins + 15 mins stretch and strengthen	Day 37 15 mins stretch and strengthen
Week 7	Day 43 Walk 14.4km (9 miles) 135–144 mins + 15 mins stretch and strengthen	Day 44 15 mins stretch and strengthen
Week 8	Day 50 15 mins stretch and strengthen	Day 51 Walk 8km (5 miles) about 75 mins + 15 mins stretch and strengthen

Other pages to help you: Using a smartphone and apps, see p52 • Treadmill walking, see pp124–125 • Nordic walking, see pp134–135 • Rucking, see pp130–131 • Upper and lower body stretches, see pp84–87 • Before and after walking, see pp90–93 • Leg stretches, pp78–79

Key ■ Walk days ■ Stretch and strengthen ■ Other activity days

Tuesday	Wednesday	Thursday	Friday	Saturday	Total
Day 31 15 mins stretch and strengthen	**Day 32** Walk 9.6km (6 miles) 90–96 mins + 15 mins stretch and strengthen	**Day 33** 30 mins core stability training	**Day 34** 15 mins stretch and strengthen	**Day 35** Walk 6.4km (4 miles) 60–64 mins + 15 mins stretch and strengthen	27.2km (17 miles)
Day 38 Walk 9.6km (6 miles) about 90 mins + 15 mins stretch and strengthen	**Day 39** Interval training 4.8km (3 miles) 45–50 mins + 15 mins stretch and strengthen	**Day 40** 15 mins stretch and strengthen	**Day 41** Any other activity for a minimum of 30 minutes	**Day 42** Walk 6.4km (4 miles) about 60 mins + 15 mins stretch and strengthen	33.7km (21 miles)
Day 45 Walk 8km (5 miles) 75–80 mins + 15 mins stretch and strengthen	**Day 46** Any other activity for a minimum of 30 minutes	**Day 47** 15 mins stretch and strengthen	**Day 48** Interval training 4.8km (3 miles) 45–50 mins + 15 mins stretch and strengthen	**Day 49** Walk 11.2km (7 miles) about 105 mins + 15 mins stretch and strengthen	38.4km (24 miles)
Day 52 Hill walking 4.8km (3 miles) 50–55 mins + 15 mins stretch and strengthen	**Day 53** 15 mins stretch and strengthen	**Day 54** Walk 6.4km (4 miles) 60–64 mins + 15 mins stretch and strengthen	**Day 55** 15 mins stretch and strengthen	**Day 56** Walk 14.4km (9 miles) 135–144 mins + 15 mins stretch and strengthen	33.6km (21 miles)

TRAINING PROGRAMMES 159

INTERMEDIATE WEEKS 9–12

Weeks 9–12
In these final weeks of the plan, you should feel you have reached a new level of fitness. For maintenance, you could repeat the plan by increasing the distances of the walks as well as their intensity. Increase the challenge by Nordic walking, rucking, or even interval training and take your stength and fitness to the next level. Bear in mind, though, that it is not advisable to interval train on two consecutive days.

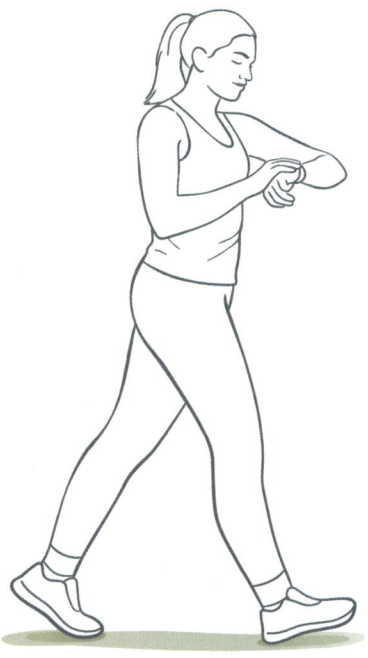

	Sunday	Monday
Week 9	**Day 57** Any other activity *for a minimum of 30 minutes*	**Day 58** 15 mins stretch and strengthen
Week 10	**Day 64** Walk 16km (10 miles) *about 150 mins + 15 mins stretch and strengthen*	**Day 65** 15 mins stretch and strengthen
Week 11	**Day 71** 15 mins stretch and strengthen	**Day 72** Walk 8km (5 miles) *75–80 mins + 15 mins stretch and strengthen*
Week 12	**Day 78** Hill walking 6.4km (4 miles) *about 60 mins + 15 mins stretch and strengthen*	**Day 79** 15 mins stretch and strengthen

Other pages to help you: Using a smartphone and apps, see p52 • Treadmill walking, see pp124–125 • Nordic walking, see pp134–135 • Rucking, see pp130–131 • Upper and lower body stretches, see pp84–87 • Before and after walking, see pp90–93 • Leg stretches, pp78–79

Key ■ Walk days   □ Stretch and strengthen   ▪ Other activity days

Tuesday	Wednesday	Thursday	Friday	Saturday	Total
Day 59 Interval training 4.8km (3 miles) *45–50 mins + 15 mins stretch and strengthen*	**Day 60** 15 mins stretch and strengthen	**Day 61** Walk 8km (5 miles) *70–75 mins + 15 mins stretch and strengthen*	**Day 62** Walk 6.4km (4 miles) *56–60 mins + 15 mins stretch and strengthen*	**Day 63** 15 mins stretch and strengthen	19.2km (12 miles)
Day 66 Interval training 6.4km (4 miles) *58–60 mins + 15 mins stretch and strengthen*	**Day 67** Walk 6.4km (4 miles) *about 60 mins + 15 mins stretch and strengthen*	**Day 68** 15 mins stretch and strengthen	**Day 69** Any other activity *for 60 minutes*	**Day 70** Walk 11.2km (7 miles) *about 98 mins + 15 mins stretch and strengthen*	40km (25 miles)
Day 73 15 mins stretch and strengthen	**Day 74** Interval training 6.4km (4 miles) *58–60 mins + 15 mins stretch and strengthen*	**Day 75** 15 mins stretch and strengthen	**Day 76** Any other activity *for 60 minutes*	**Day 77** Walk 14.4km (9 miles) *126–135 mins + 15 mins stretch and strengthen*	28.8km (18 miles)
Day 80 Walk 9.6km (6 miles) *84–90 mins + 15 mins stretch and strengthen*	**Day 81** Core stability training *for 60 mins*	**Day 82** Walk 4.8km (3 miles) *39–42 mins + 15 mins stretch and strengthen*	**Day 83** 15 mins stretch and strengthen	**Day 84** Walk 16km (10 miles) *140–150 mins + 15 mins stretch and strengthen*	36.8km (23 miles)

Full marathon

LEVEL: 3 / TOTAL: 12 WEEKS

There can be many reasons for taking on a marathon, from achieving a personal goal, to raising money for charity. Whatever the aim, that moment of crossing the finish line is magical. By following this 12-week plan the magic could be yours!

WEEKS 1–4

A good finishing time for power walking a marathon (42.2km/26¼ miles) is 6 hours. Aim to walk at a constant speed of 12–14 minutes per 1.6km (1 mile).

Weeks 1–2
In these first weeks, work on your technique and posture. Exert yourself beyond your normal walking speed, feeling an increase in your heart rate, while keeping the pace constant. Going too fast too soon will feel uncomfortable and can cause injuries. Start with around 10 minutes and extend this as you are ready. Always warm up and cool down for each session. On the days when you are not walking, set aside time for stretching and strengthening, and don't forget about your AM–PM (the steps you take from getting up to going to bed).

Week 3
By now you need to be increasing your pace. Although you are exerting yourself, make sure you are still able to talk as you walk. The other activity can be anything you enjoy, such as swimming, dancing, or Pilates.

Week 4
Whille increasing your pace, introduce interval training into your mid-week sessions. It works the body quite hard, so take it steady, have a rest day afterwards or an easy walk.

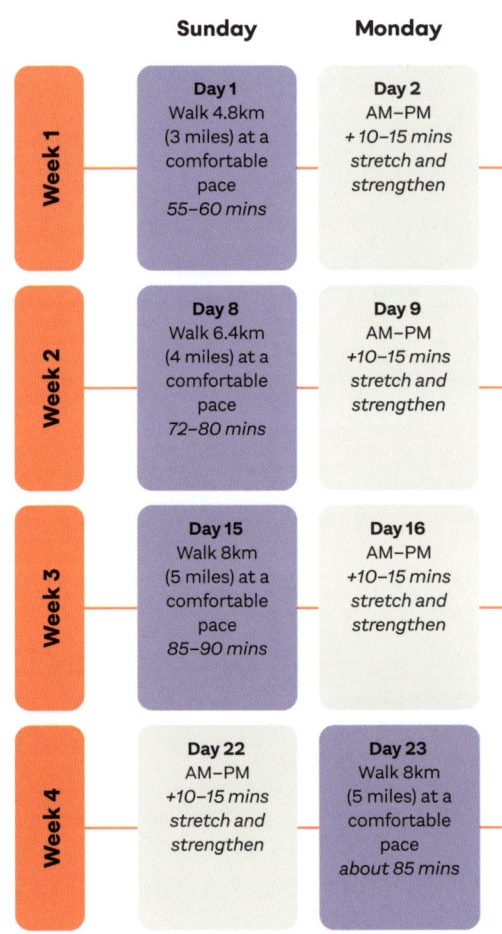

For this programme, you must be able to walk 4.8km (3 miles) at a steady spead of approximately 18–20 minutes per 1.6km (1 mile). If you can't yet reach this pace, follow the Beginner programme until you can, then return to this one. Marathon training should always be on tarmac or even surfaces.

Other pages to help you: Using a smartphone and apps, see p52 • Interval training, see pp122-123 • Foods for health and fitness, see pp116–119 • Warming up and cooling down, see pp90–93 • Stretch and strengthen routine, see p95 • Cross training, see pp180-181 • Competitive race walking, see pp136–137

Key Walk days   Stretch and strengthen   Other activity days

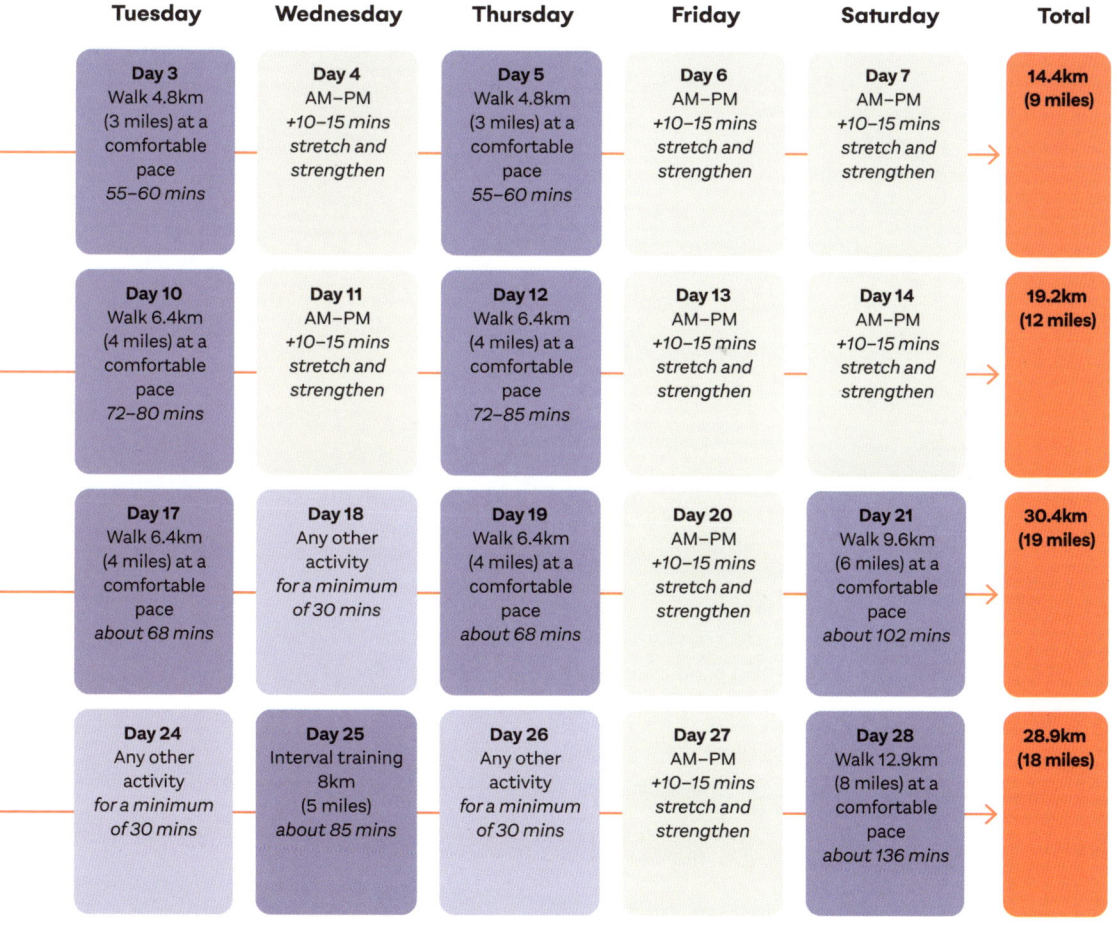

Tuesday	Wednesday	Thursday	Friday	Saturday	Total
Day 3 Walk 4.8km (3 miles) at a comfortable pace *55–60 mins*	**Day 4** AM–PM *+10–15 mins stretch and strengthen*	**Day 5** Walk 4.8km (3 miles) at a comfortable pace *55–60 mins*	**Day 6** AM–PM *+10–15 mins stretch and strengthen*	**Day 7** AM–PM *+10–15 mins stretch and strengthen*	**14.4km (9 miles)**
Day 10 Walk 6.4km (4 miles) at a comfortable pace *72–80 mins*	**Day 11** AM–PM *+10–15 mins stretch and strengthen*	**Day 12** Walk 6.4km (4 miles) at a comfortable pace *72–85 mins*	**Day 13** AM–PM *+10–15 mins stretch and strengthen*	**Day 14** AM–PM *+10–15 mins stretch and strengthen*	**19.2km (12 miles)**
Day 17 Walk 6.4km (4 miles) at a comfortable pace *about 68 mins*	**Day 18** Any other activity *for a minimum of 30 mins*	**Day 19** Walk 6.4km (4 miles) at a comfortable pace *about 68 mins*	**Day 20** AM–PM *+10–15 mins stretch and strengthen*	**Day 21** Walk 9.6km (6 miles) at a comfortable pace *about 102 mins*	**30.4km (19 miles)**
Day 24 Any other activity *for a minimum of 30 mins*	**Day 25** Interval training 8km (5 miles) *about 85 mins*	**Day 26** Any other activity *for a minimum of 30 mins*	**Day 27** AM–PM *+10–15 mins stretch and strengthen*	**Day 28** Walk 12.9km (8 miles) at a comfortable pace *about 136 mins*	**28.9km (18 miles)**

FULL MARATHON WEEKS 5–8

Weeks 5–8
By week 5 you should be starting to feel the physical and mental benefits as you get into the rhythm of regular walking. It's important to track your progress of how feel, as well as how far you walk and at what pace.

Once a week, try introducing some interval training. Alternate between walking as fast as you can for 1–2 minutes and then slowing down to recover for double the time of your fast walk, (2–4 minutes). You can repeat this as often as you wish, but take it steady, as it is an intense form of training. Only do the amount that feels comfortable, building up slowly. Don't forget to celebrate each stepping stone of success, no matter how small – these small steps are a huge motivation to keep going!

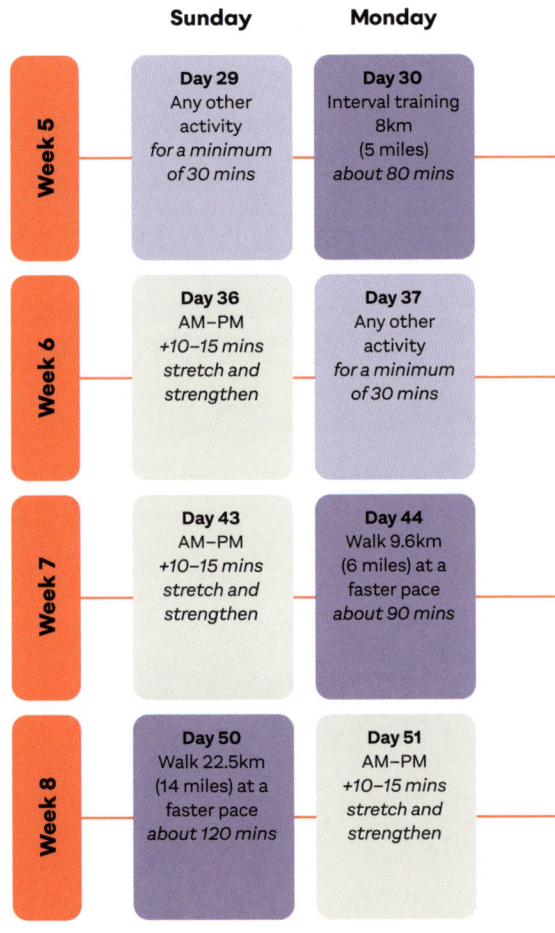

	Sunday	Monday
Week 5	**Day 29** Any other activity *for a minimum of 30 mins*	**Day 30** Interval training 8km (5 miles) *about 80 mins*
Week 6	**Day 36** AM–PM *+10–15 mins stretch and strengthen*	**Day 37** Any other activity *for a minimum of 30 mins*
Week 7	**Day 43** AM–PM *+10–15 mins stretch and strengthen*	**Day 44** Walk 9.6km (6 miles) at a faster pace *about 90 mins*
Week 8	**Day 50** Walk 22.5km (14 miles) at a faster pace *about 120 mins*	**Day 51** AM–PM *+10–15 mins stretch and strengthen*

"Don't forget to celebrate each stepping stone of success, no matter how small."

164   WALK YOURSELF WELL

Other pages to help you: Using a smartphone and apps, see p52 • Interval training, see pp122–123 • Foods for health and fitness, see pp116–119 • Warming up and cooling down, see pp90–93 • Stretch and strengthen routine, see p95 • Cross training, see pp180–181 • Competitive race walking, see pp136–137

Key: Walk days | Stretch and strengthen | Other activity days

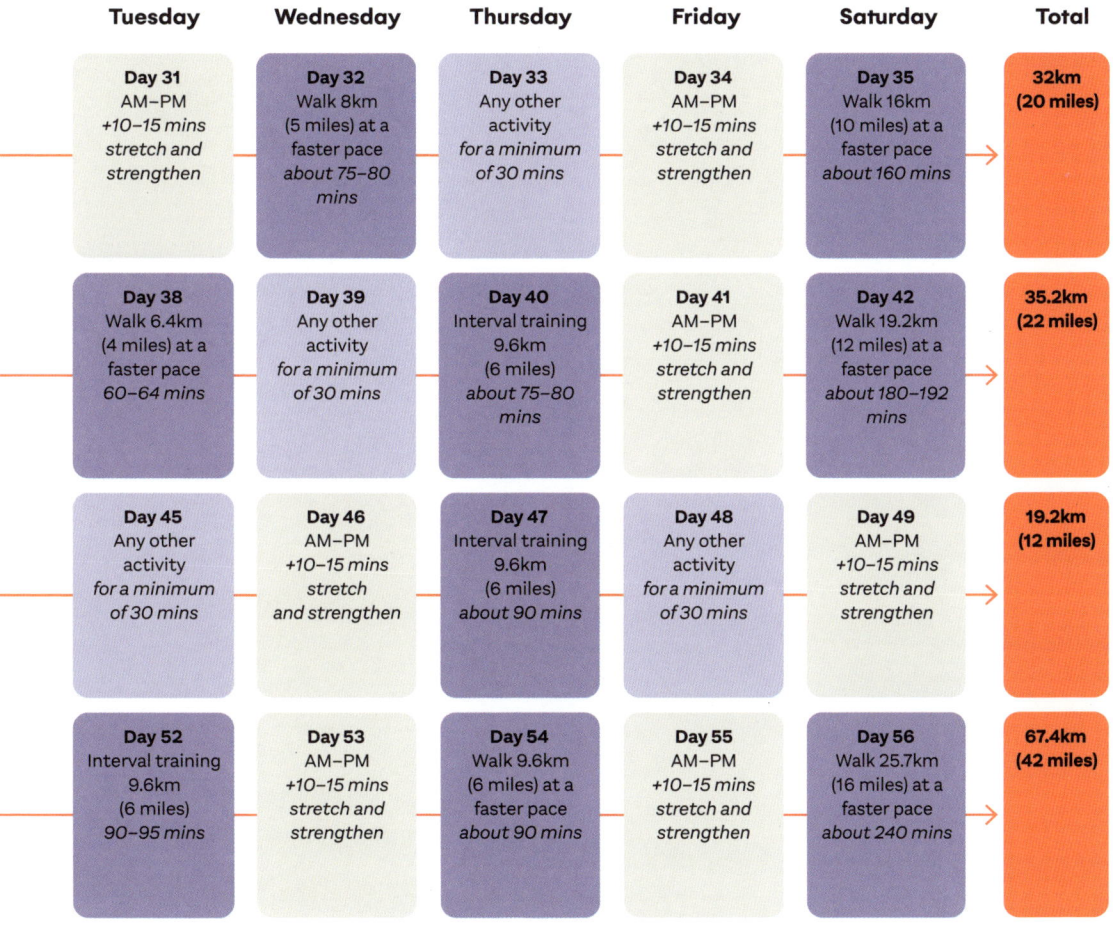

Tuesday	Wednesday	Thursday	Friday	Saturday	Total
Day 31 AM–PM +10–15 mins stretch and strengthen	**Day 32** Walk 8km (5 miles) at a faster pace about 75–80 mins	**Day 33** Any other activity for a minimum of 30 mins	**Day 34** AM–PM +10–15 mins stretch and strengthen	**Day 35** Walk 16km (10 miles) at a faster pace about 160 mins	**32km (20 miles)**
Day 38 Walk 6.4km (4 miles) at a faster pace 60–64 mins	**Day 39** Any other activity for a minimum of 30 mins	**Day 40** Interval training 9.6km (6 miles) about 75–80 mins	**Day 41** AM–PM +10–15 mins stretch and strengthen	**Day 42** Walk 19.2km (12 miles) at a faster pace about 180–192 mins	**35.2km (22 miles)**
Day 45 Any other activity for a minimum of 30 mins	**Day 46** AM–PM +10–15 mins stretch and strengthen	**Day 47** Interval training 9.6km (6 miles) about 90 mins	**Day 48** Any other activity for a minimum of 30 mins	**Day 49** AM–PM +10–15 mins stretch and strengthen	**19.2km (12 miles)**
Day 52 Interval training 9.6km (6 miles) 90–95 mins	**Day 53** AM–PM +10–15 mins stretch and strengthen	**Day 54** Walk 9.6km (6 miles) at a faster pace about 90 mins	**Day 55** AM–PM +10–15 mins stretch and strengthen	**Day 56** Walk 25.7km (16 miles) at a faster pace about 240 mins	**67.4km (42 miles)**

TRAINING PROGRAMMES

FULL MARATHON WEEKS 9–12

Weeks 9–12
In the final 4 weeks of the plan you will not only reach the climax of your training, but also head into a rest period following your 32km (20 mile) walk, allowing your body recovery time prior to the challenge.

Walking the 32km (20 mile) distance is an important part of the plan, both mentally and physically. If you can complete this distance, you can be confident that you'll reach the finish line. If you have not done so already, take the opportunity in these last few weeks to eat well, stay hydrated, and commit to spending time each day stretching. This level of preparation will contribute to how supported your body feels on the day.

Don't forget that post-event care is also important. Your body will probably have been running on adrenalin for quite some time. As soon as you cross the finish line, eat proteins and carbohydrates to replenish your blood sugar levels and muscle glycogen to help repair muscle tissue. Hot soup is comforting if the weather is cold – otherwise porridge, a peanut butter sandwich, or yogurt with cereal are all good choices.

Make sure you have something warm to put on. Although you may not feel like it, slowly keep walking to release the lactic acid from your muscles. Of course, stretching on the day and subsequent days following the challenge is a must! Good luck.

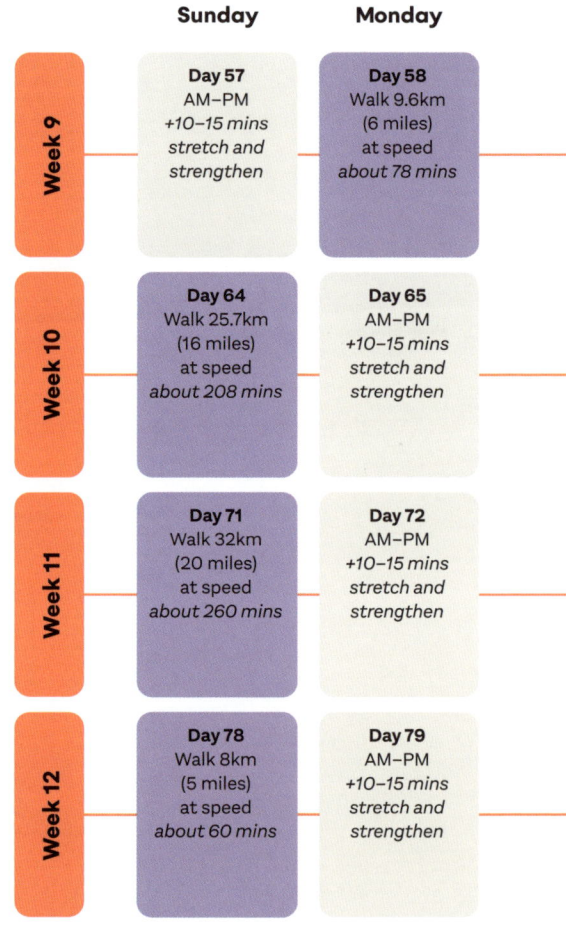

	Sunday	Monday
Week 9	Day 57 AM–PM +10–15 mins stretch and strengthen	Day 58 Walk 9.6km (6 miles) at speed about 78 mins
Week 10	Day 64 Walk 25.7km (16 miles) at speed about 208 mins	Day 65 AM–PM +10–15 mins stretch and strengthen
Week 11	Day 71 Walk 32km (20 miles) at speed about 260 mins	Day 72 AM–PM +10–15 mins stretch and strengthen
Week 12	Day 78 Walk 8km (5 miles) at speed about 60 mins	Day 79 AM–PM +10–15 mins stretch and strengthen

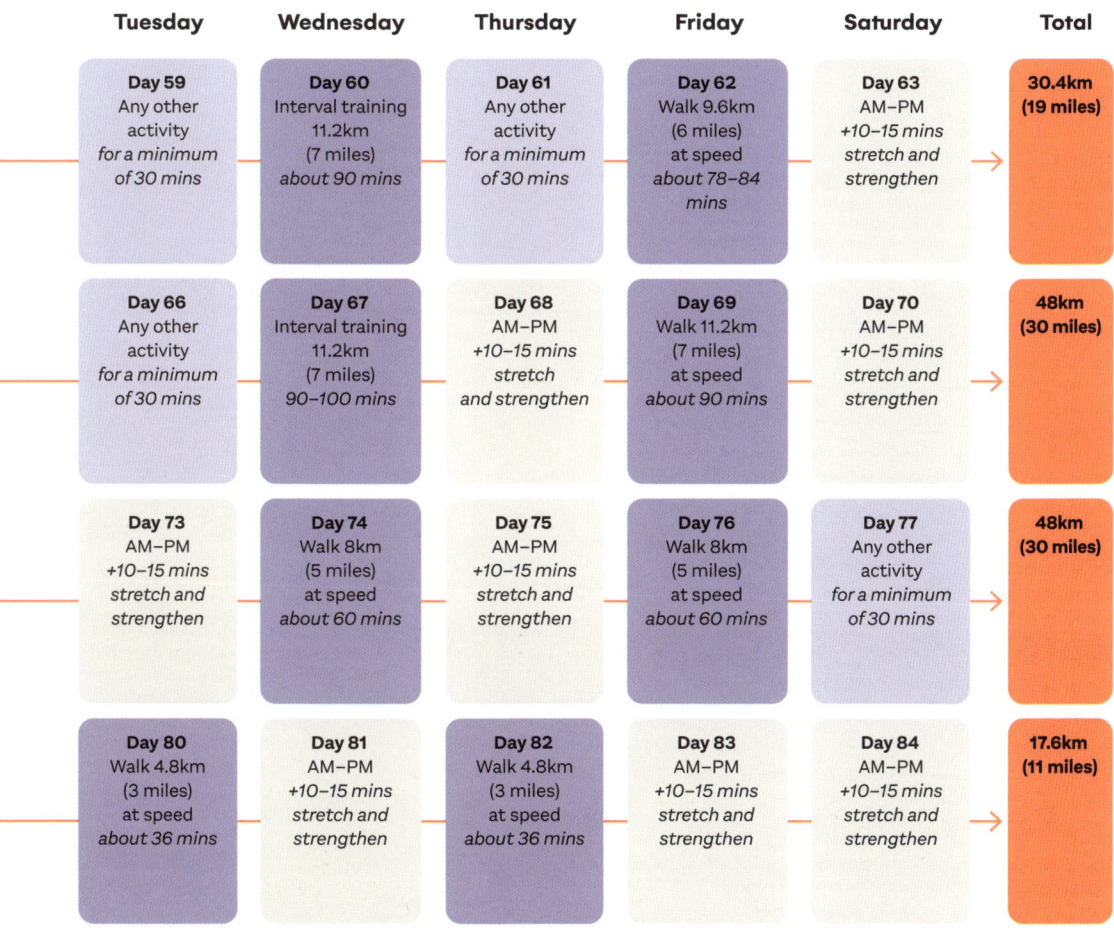

Other pages to help you: Using a smartphone and apps, see p52 • Interval training, see pp122-123 • Foods for health and fitness, see pp116–119 • Warming up and cooling down, see pp90–93 • Stretch and strengthen routine, see p95 • Cross training, see pp180–181 • Competitive race walking, see pp136–137

TRAINING PROGRAMMES 167

Advanced: long distances, hikes, and challenges

LEVEL: 3 / TOTAL: 12 WEEKS

This programme is for walkers wanting to add distance and intensity to their walking. There are three stages: the first builds stamina, the second focuses on speed, and the third brings both aspects together to help you achieve a high level of ability. Your aim is to sustain a walking speed of 12–13 minutes per 1.6km (1 mile).

WEEKS 1–4

Before you start this programme you must be able to walk 1.6km (1 mile) in 15 minutes at a constant pace, and walk comfortably for 16km (10 miles) at a reasonable pace. You can repeat any part of the programme until you are ready to move on to the next stage. Setting both a distance to walk and an ideal speed in which to complete it, and walking to the speed suggested for each kilometre (or mile), you will progress quickly. However, always match the intensity of your walk to what you feel you can manage on a given day. A training walk can be exchanged for working with weights for 30 minutes or a walk on a treadmill, but ideally not more than once a week.

Weeks 1–4
During these weeks you are building stamina and strength with daily stretching, core stability exercises, and long-distance walks. Developing strong core muscles is key to walking at speed. To expand the sequence for the stretching times specified, hold your form for longer and add more repetitions. Including interval training can also add a new dimension. This is an intense workout, so only complete it 1–2 times a week and follow with an easy workout or rest the next day. Hill walking and even rucking can all add variety.

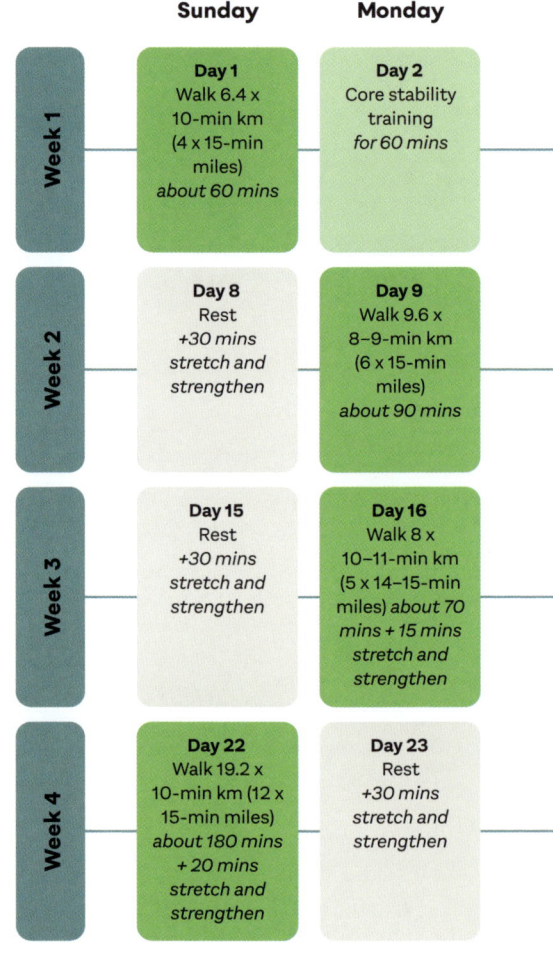

	Sunday	**Monday**
Week 1	**Day 1** Walk 6.4 x 10-min km (4 x 15-min miles) about 60 mins	**Day 2** Core stability training *for 60 mins*
Week 2	**Day 8** Rest *+30 mins stretch and strengthen*	**Day 9** Walk 9.6 x 8–9-min km (6 x 15-min miles) about 90 mins
Week 3	**Day 15** Rest *+30 mins stretch and strengthen*	**Day 16** Walk 8 x 10–11-min km (5 x 14–15-min miles) about 70 mins + 15 mins stretch and strengthen
Week 4	**Day 22** Walk 19.2 x 10-min km (12 x 15-min miles) about 180 mins + 20 mins stretch and strengthen	**Day 23** Rest *+30 mins stretch and strengthen*

You will be working your body both aerobically and anaerobically. By using a heart-rate monitor you can balance time and intensity to work within your optimum levels. If you are short of time, concentrate on walking fast shorter distances, or intervals. Variety is key to motivation.

Other pages to help you: Interval training, see pp122–123 • Staying injury-free, see pp70–73 • Nordic walking, see pp134–135 • Rucking, see pp130–131 • Before and after walking, see pp90–93 • Foods for health and fitness, see pp116–119 • Warming up and cooling down, see pp90–93 • Stretch and strengthen routine, see p95 • Core training, see pp80–83 • Cross training, see pp180–181

Key ■ Walk days ▫ Rest days ■ Other activity days

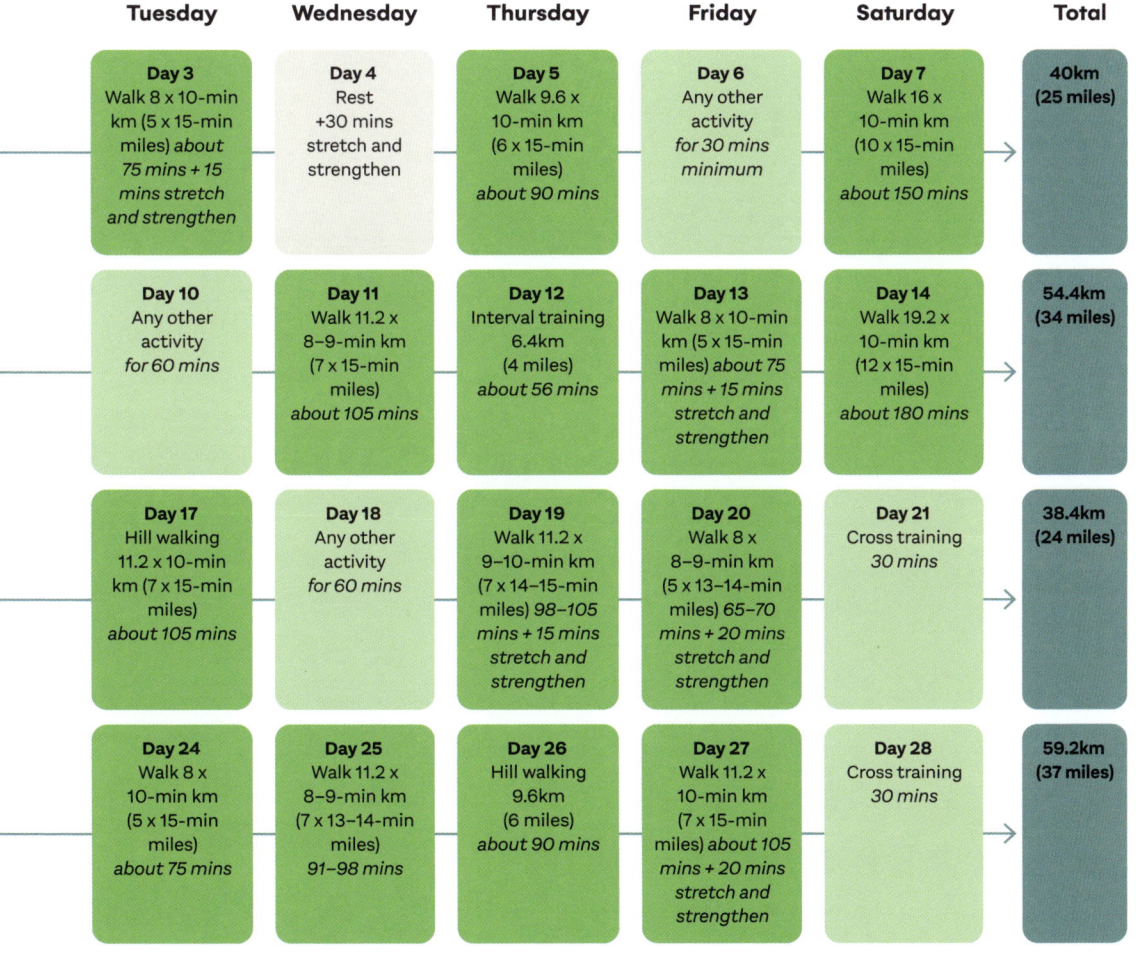

	Tuesday	Wednesday	Thursday	Friday	Saturday	Total
	Day 3 Walk 8 x 10-min km (5 x 15-min miles) about 75 mins + 15 mins stretch and strengthen	**Day 4** Rest +30 mins stretch and strengthen	**Day 5** Walk 9.6 x 10-min km (6 x 15-min miles) about 90 mins	**Day 6** Any other activity for 30 mins minimum	**Day 7** Walk 16 x 10-min km (10 x 15-min miles) about 150 mins	40km (25 miles)
	Day 10 Any other activity for 60 mins	**Day 11** Walk 11.2 x 8–9-min km (7 x 15-min miles) about 105 mins	**Day 12** Interval training 6.4km (4 miles) about 56 mins	**Day 13** Walk 8 x 10-min km (5 x 15-min miles) about 75 mins + 15 mins stretch and strengthen	**Day 14** Walk 19.2 x 10-min km (12 x 15-min miles) about 180 mins	54.4km (34 miles)
	Day 17 Hill walking 11.2 x 10-min km (7 x 15-min miles) about 105 mins	**Day 18** Any other activity for 60 mins	**Day 19** Walk 11.2 x 9–10-min km (7 x 14–15-min miles) 98–105 mins + 15 mins stretch and strengthen	**Day 20** Walk 8 x 8–9-min km (5 x 13–14-min miles) 65–70 mins + 20 mins stretch and strengthen	**Day 21** Cross training 30 mins	38.4km (24 miles)
	Day 24 Walk 8 x 10-min km (5 x 15-min miles) about 75 mins	**Day 25** Walk 11.2 x 8–9-min km (7 x 13–14-min miles) 91–98 mins	**Day 26** Hill walking 9.6km (6 miles) about 90 mins	**Day 27** Walk 11.2 x 10-min km (7 x 15-min miles) about 105 mins + 20 mins stretch and strengthen	**Day 28** Cross training 30 mins	59.2km (37 miles)

TRAINING PROGRAMMES 169

ADVANCED WEEKS 5–8

Weeks 5–8
The focus for the next 4 weeks is to work on walking shorter distances, but with increased intensity and speed. It is advisable to keep to roads, pavements, or flat surfaces for this part of the plan.

The combination of walking, interval training, and core stability work is an ideal way to increase overall body strength, muscle tone, and fitness. By this point, you should already be feeling a difference in your physical ability.

Kettlebells are an ideal discipline to include in your training, providing a versatile range of exercises that not only engage your core, but multiple other muscle groups. They are particularly good at developing hip strength, stability, and balance, and for building endurance and overall body power. It is important to join a class initially to have lessons from a qualified instructor, as good technique is essential. After that you can easily do your sessions at home.

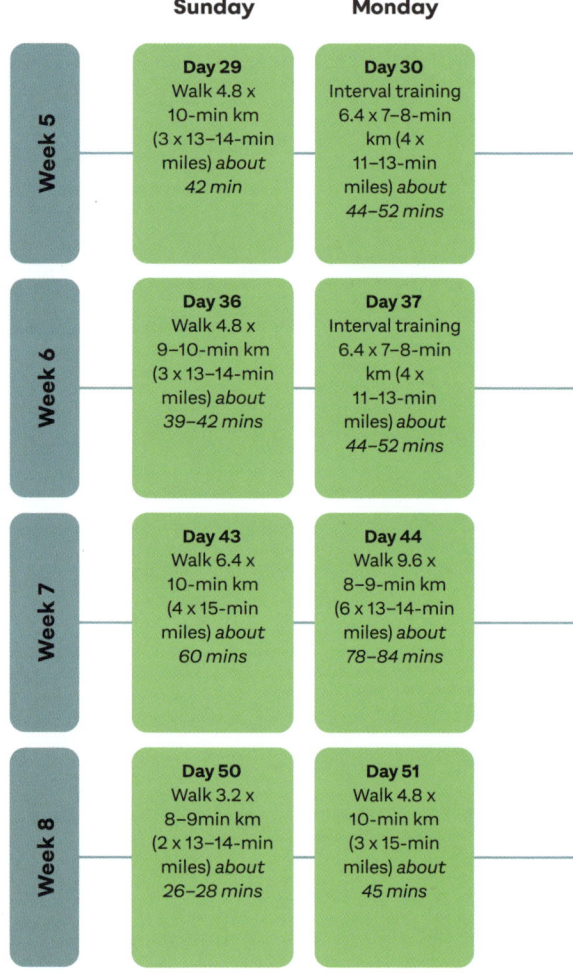

	Sunday	Monday
Week 5	**Day 29** Walk 4.8 x 10-min km (3 x 13–14-min miles) *about 42 min*	**Day 30** Interval training 6.4 x 7–8-min km (4 x 11–13-min miles) *about 44–52 mins*
Week 6	**Day 36** Walk 4.8 x 9–10-min km (3 x 13–14-min miles) *about 39–42 mins*	**Day 37** Interval training 6.4 x 7–8-min km (4 x 11–13-min miles) *about 44–52 mins*
Week 7	**Day 43** Walk 6.4 x 10-min km (4 x 15-min miles) *about 60 mins*	**Day 44** Walk 9.6 x 8–9-min km (6 x 13–14-min miles) *about 78–84 mins*
Week 8	**Day 50** Walk 3.2 x 8–9min km (2 x 13–14-min miles) *about 26–28 mins*	**Day 51** Walk 4.8 x 10-min km (3 x 15-min miles) *about 45 mins*

Other pages to help you: Interval training, see pp122–123 • Staying injury-free, see pp70–73 • Nordic walking, see pp134–135 • Rucking, see pp130–131 • Before and after walking, see pp90–93 • Foods for health and fitness, see pp116–119 • Warming up and cooling down, see pp90–93 • Stretch and strengthen routine, see p95 • Core training, see pp80–83 • Cross training, see pp180–181

Key ■ Walk days   □ Rest days   ■ Other activity days

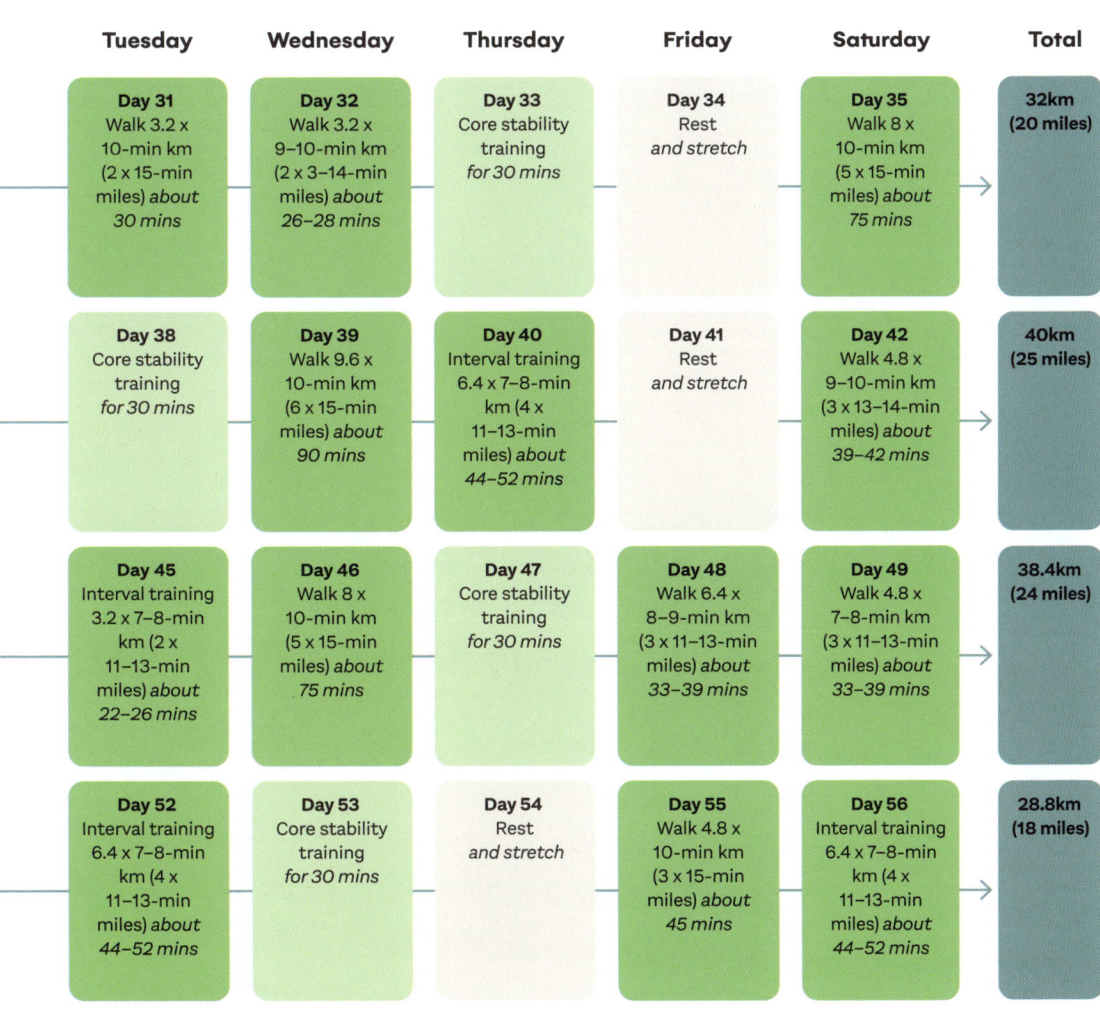

Tuesday	Wednesday	Thursday	Friday	Saturday	Total
Day 31 Walk 3.2 x 10-min km (2 x 15-min miles) *about 30 mins*	**Day 32** Walk 3.2 x 9–10-min km (2 x 3–14-min miles) *about 26–28 mins*	**Day 33** Core stability training *for 30 mins*	**Day 34** Rest *and stretch*	**Day 35** Walk 8 x 10-min km (5 x 15-min miles) *about 75 mins*	32km (20 miles)
Day 38 Core stability training *for 30 mins*	**Day 39** Walk 9.6 x 10-min km (6 x 15-min miles) *about 90 mins*	**Day 40** Interval training 6.4 x 7–8-min km (4 x 11–13-min miles) *about 44–52 mins*	**Day 41** Rest *and stretch*	**Day 42** Walk 4.8 x 9–10-min km (3 x 13–14-min miles) *about 39–42 mins*	40km (25 miles)
Day 45 Interval training 3.2 x 7–8-min km (2 x 11–13-min miles) *about 22–26 mins*	**Day 46** Walk 8 x 10-min km (5 x 15-min miles) *about 75 mins*	**Day 47** Core stability training *for 30 mins*	**Day 48** Walk 6.4 x 8–9-min km (3 x 11–13-min miles) *about 33–39 mins*	**Day 49** Walk 4.8 x 7–8-min km (3 x 11–13-min miles) *about 33–39 mins*	38.4km (24 miles)
Day 52 Interval training 6.4 x 7–8-min km (4 x 11–13-min miles) *about 44–52 mins*	**Day 53** Core stability training *for 30 mins*	**Day 54** Rest *and stretch*	**Day 55** Walk 4.8 x 10-min km (3 x 15-min miles) *about 45 mins*	**Day 56** Interval training 6.4 x 7–8-min km (4 x 11–13-min miles) *about 44–52 mins*	28.8km (18 miles)

ADVANCED WEEKS 9-12

Weeks 9-12
The final 4 weeks of the plan is a process of bringing together all the technique and skills that you have worked on, to be able to walk with speed and stamina.

When you have completed the plan you can use the programme as a guide or as a base to create your own. Continue increasing the distance and speed depending on your goal. Keep exploring new routes that test your ability and help to keep you motivated.

You now have a good fitness level to explore taking on a new challenge. Whether it is a long-distance trek, cross-country Nordic walking, rucking, or even a marathon that you want to complete in a good finishing time, you have the power, endurance, and strength – the choice is yours!

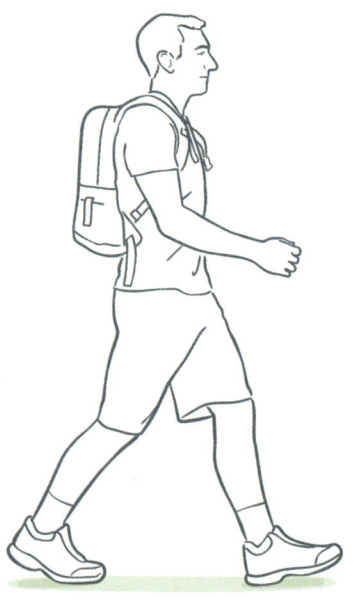

	Sunday	Monday
Week 9	**Day 57** Any other activity *for a minimum of 30 minutes*	**Day 58** Interval training 6.4km (4 miles) *48-54 mins*
Week 10	**Day 64** Walk 8 x 9-min km (5 x 14-min miles) *about 70 mins + 20 mins stretch and strengthen*	**Day 65** Walk 11.2 x 8-9-min km (7 x 12-14-min miles) *about 84-98 mins*
Week 11	**Day 71** Walk 19.2 x 8-10-min km (12 x 13-14-min miles) *156-168 mins + 20 mins stretch and strengthen*	**Day 72** Core stability training *for 30 mins*
Week 12	**Day 78** Walk 6.4 x 10-min km (4 x 15-min miles) *about 60 mins*	**Day 79** Walk 8 x 7-8-min km (5 x 11-13-min miles) *55-56 mins + 15 mins stretch and strengthen*

Other pages to help you: Interval training, see pp122–123 • Staying injury-free, see pp70–73 • Nordic walking, see pp134–135 • Rucking, see pp130–131 • Before and after walking, see pp90–93 • Foods for health and fitness, see pp116–119 • Warming up and cooling down, see pp90–93 • Stretch and strengthen routine, see p95 • Core training, see pp80–83 • Cross training, see pp180–181

Key ▇ Walk days ▢ Rest days ▇ Other activity days

Tuesday	Wednesday	Thursday	Friday	Saturday	Total
Day 59 Walk 9.6 x 7–8-min km (6 x 11–13-min miles) 66–78 mins	**Day 60** Core stability training *for 30 mins*	**Day 61** Walk 4.8 x 8-min km (3 x 13-min miles) *about 36 mins*	**Day 62** Hill walking 6.4km (4 miles) 52–60 mins	**Day 63** Walk 16 x 9–10-min km (10 x 13–15-min miles) 130–150 mins	43.2km (27 miles)
Day 66 Core stability training *for 30 mins*	**Day 67** Rest *and stretch*	**Day 68** Hill walking 6.4km (4 miles) *about 48–52 mins + 15 mins stretch and strengthen*	**Day 69** Interval training 9.6km (6 miles) *about 78–84 mins + 20 mins stretch and strengthen*	**Day 70** Walk 11.2 x 7–8-min km (7 x 12–14-min miles) *about 84–98 mins + 15 mins stretch and strengthen*	46.4km (29 miles)
Day 73 Walk 4.8 x 7-min km (3 x 11-min miles) *about 33 mins + 20 mins stretch and strengthen*	**Day 74** Walk 8 x 9-min km (5 x 14-min miles) *about 70 mins + 15 mins stretch and strengthen*	**Day 75** Rest *and stretch*	**Day 76** Walk 9.6 x 8-min km (6 x 11–13-min miles) 66–78 *mins + 20 mins stretch and strengthen*	**Day 77** Hill walking 16 x 8–9-min km (10 x 13–14-min miles) 130–140 mins	57.6km (36 miles)
Day 80 Any other activity *for 60 minutes*	**Day 81** Interval training 4.8 km (3 miles) 33–39 mins	**Day 82** Core stability training *for 30 mins*	**Day 83** Walk 8 x 10-min km (5 x 15-min miles) *about 75 mins + 15 mins stretch and strengthen*	**Day 84** Walk 19.2 x 7–8-min km (12 x 11–13-min miles) 132–143 mins	46.4km (29 miles)

TRAINING PROGRAMMES 173

Ultra fitness

LEVEL: 4 / TOTAL: 12 WEEKS

The intensity of training to reach the required fitness level for an extreme or ultra challenge of any distance demands dedicated commitment. You will be placing a significant pressure on yourself for both time, and physical effort. But, if you prepare, the reward is thrilling and definitely worth reaching for.

WEEKS 1–4

It is worth noting that for those wanting to achieve the required starting fitness, or for those taking on 100km challenge or back-to-back consecutive marathons, it is advisable to add a further 4 weeks onto your training plan to allow more time to reach your peak. Also consider a longer pre-event walk if you are walking further than 42km (26 miles). With any intense training, it is important to always be aware of how you feel. If at any point you feel uncomfortable or unwell, consult medical advice immediately.

Weeks 1–4
Use these weeks to establish a routine, once you find the space in your life to fit in the miles and activities, which can be challenging. Put training sessions in your diary as appointments that you are less likely to change. Although the plan and activities are set week by week, you can change them to suit your life, as long as the total sessions each week are the same. Book an assessment with a personal trainer, try different activities, use cross training equipment, and discover what you like. It's not important that you stick to the same activities throughout, but it does initially help in creating a routine. There is a lot to think about, so the more streamlined you can make it, the better.

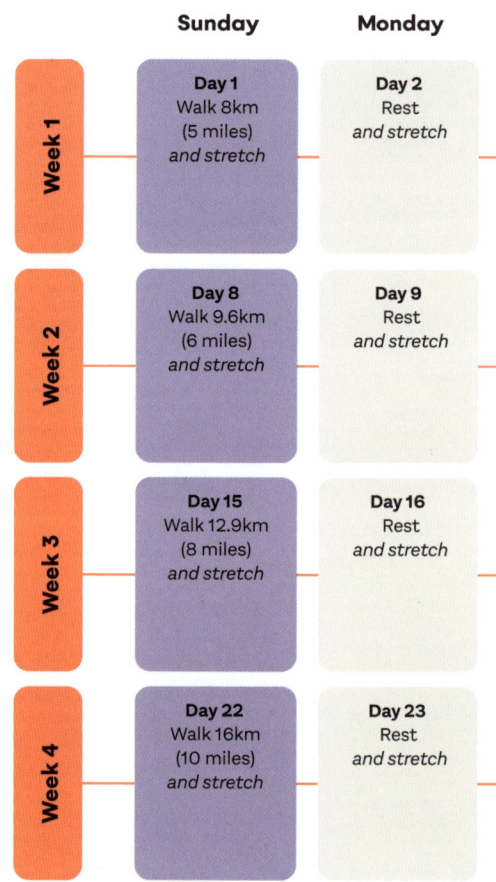

The aim is to build total body strength, stamina, and fitness that will allow you to complete an ultra or extreme walking challenge. The plan assumes you have a good level of fitness and can comfortably walk 6.5km (4 miles) at a 14–15 minute per 1.6km (1 mile) pace. Emphasis is also placed on including cross training and other activities to help develop the all-round strength that is required. If you are uncertain about your starting fitness, begin with a plan that will work with your current ability, and go from there.

Other pages to help you: Interval training, see pp122–123 • Foods for health and fitness, see pp116–119 • Warming up and cooling down, see pp90–93 • Stretch and strengthen routine, see p95 • Cross training, see pp180-181 • Competitive race walking, see pp136–137 • Marathons, see pp162–167

Key 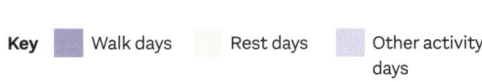 Walk days   Rest days   Other activity days

Tuesday	Wednesday	Thursday	Friday	Saturday	Total
Day 3 Cross training or any other activity 30–45 mins *Try something new!*	**Day 4** Walk 8km (5 miles) *and stretch*	**Day 5** Rest *and stretch*	**Day 6** Walk 8km (5 miles) *and stretch*	**Day 7** Swim, Pilates, or weights	**24km (15 miles)**
Day 10 Cross training or any other activity 30–45 mins *Try Pilates or kettlebell*	**Day 11** Walk 9.6km (6 miles) *and stretch*	**Day 12** Rest *and stretch*	**Day 13** Walk 9.6km (6 miles) *and stretch*	**Day 14** Swim, Pilates, or weights	**28.6km (18 miles)**
Day 17 Cross training or any other activity 30–45 mins *Try swimming or Pilates*	**Day 18** Walk 9.6km (6 miles) *and stretch Try some hills or an incline on a treadmill*	**Day 19** Rest *and stretch*	**Day 20** Walk 9.6km (6 miles) *and stretch*	**Day 21** Swim, Pilates, or weights	**32km (20 miles)**
Day 24 Cross training or any other activity 45 mins	**Day 25** Walk 9.6km (6 miles) *and stretch Don't forget to choose different routes!*	**Day 26** Rest *and stretch*	**Day 27** Walk 12.9km (8 miles) *and stretch*	**Day 28** Swim, Pilates, or weights	**38.5km (24 miles)**

ULTRA FITNESS WEEKS 5-8

Weeks 5-6
As distances begin to increase over the next 2 weeks, use this time to work on developing your technique – it will be impossible to reach the speeds you are aiming for without streamlining your body and using powerful arms to their full potential to propel yourself forwards.

A common mistake made by many is to skip stretching, whether it is before, during, or after your walk, or on your rest days. Don't underestimate the benefits you will feel and gain from making this part of your daily routine. Commit to stretching properly and, once you feel the benefits, you'll never look back!

Due to the increase in mileage, you may also want to consider alternating between two pairs of shoes, so that if it does rain you always have dry shoes.

Weeks 7-8
Your body can only perform well if it's fuelled by energy-sustaining foods and kept hydrated. You will be out walking for many hours, so increasing your water intake should start in the early stages of training. Allowing your body time to become used to the extra liquid is an important part of your preparation.

With the increased distances, you will also find your appetite increases quite considerably, so there's a great temptation to eat whatever you can lay your hands on first. Carry healthy snacks, and make sure you have satisfying easy-to-make, or pre-prepared meals in the fridge.

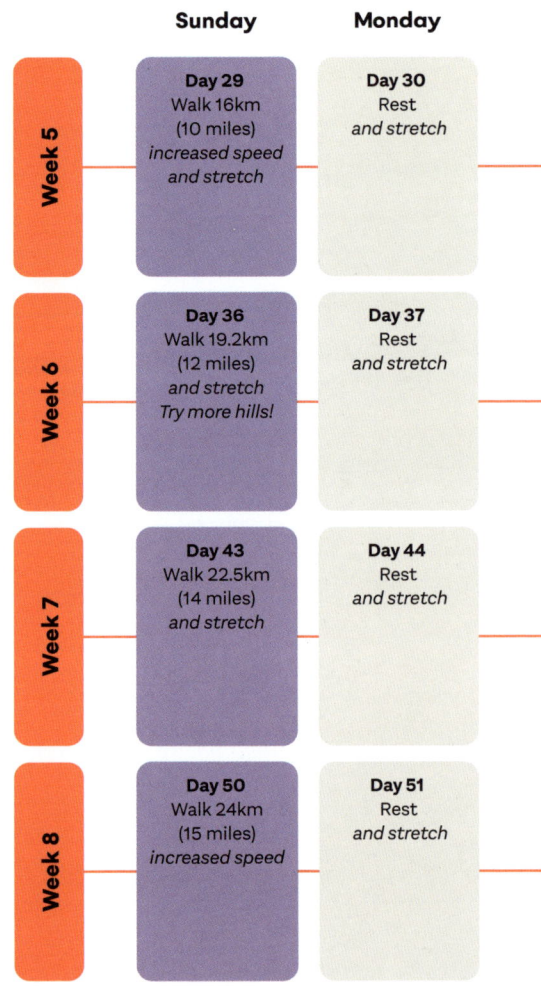

	Sunday	Monday
Week 5	**Day 29** Walk 16km (10 miles) *increased speed and stretch*	**Day 30** Rest *and stretch*
Week 6	**Day 36** Walk 19.2km (12 miles) *and stretch Try more hills!*	**Day 37** Rest *and stretch*
Week 7	**Day 43** Walk 22.5km (14 miles) *and stretch*	**Day 44** Rest *and stretch*
Week 8	**Day 50** Walk 24km (15 miles) *increased speed*	**Day 51** Rest *and stretch*

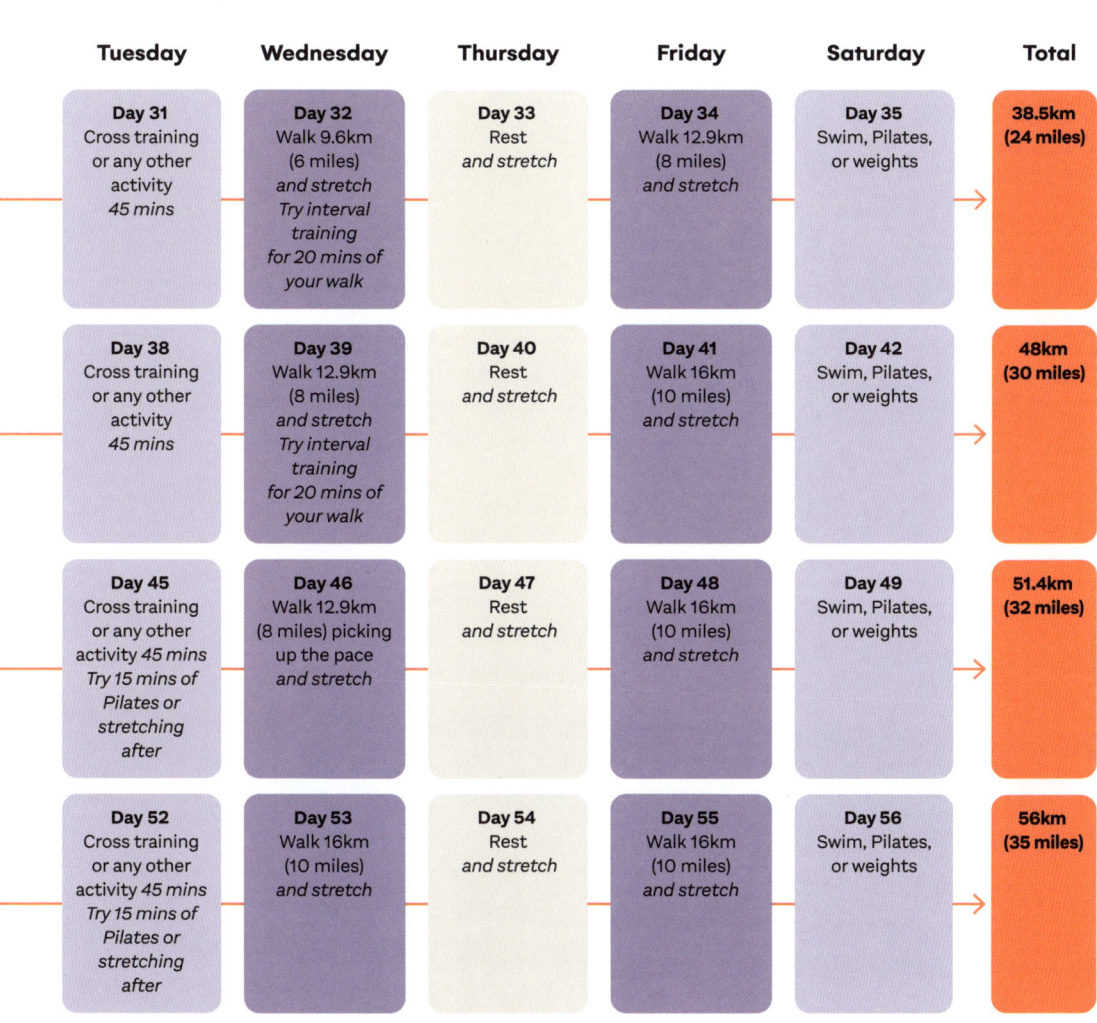

ULTRA FITNESS WEEKS 9–12

Weeks 9–12
Don't forget to regularly alternate and change your routes so they are fresh and interesting. This plays a big part in staying motivated, especially on long distances.

Your training climax comes 2 weeks before your challenge – or start day if you are trekking. By now you should feel strong, and very much in control of your physical fitness. Whatever your intended goal, completing this plan is an important step towards mental and physical confidence and endurance.

From your Week 10 or Week 12 long walk, depending on your plan, reduce all distances to a maintenance level, as it will take your body approximately 2 weeks to recover. Help it along with plenty of good food, relaxation, stretching, and sleep.

Use visualization to picture yourself achieving your goal, or crossing the finish line and receiving your medal. Over 50 per cent of a challenge is mental, so if you think you can you will, and if you think you can't you won't!

> "Use visualization to picture yourself crossing the finish line and receiving your medal."

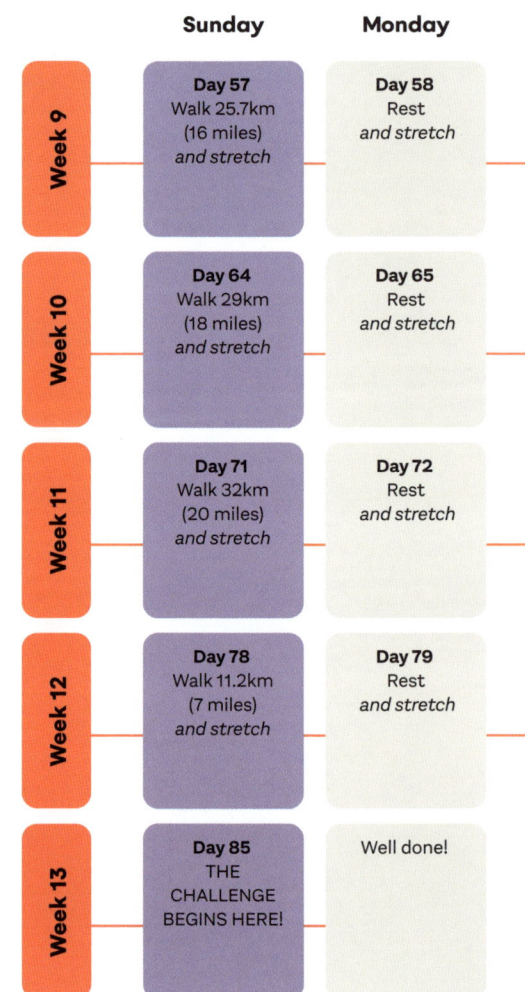

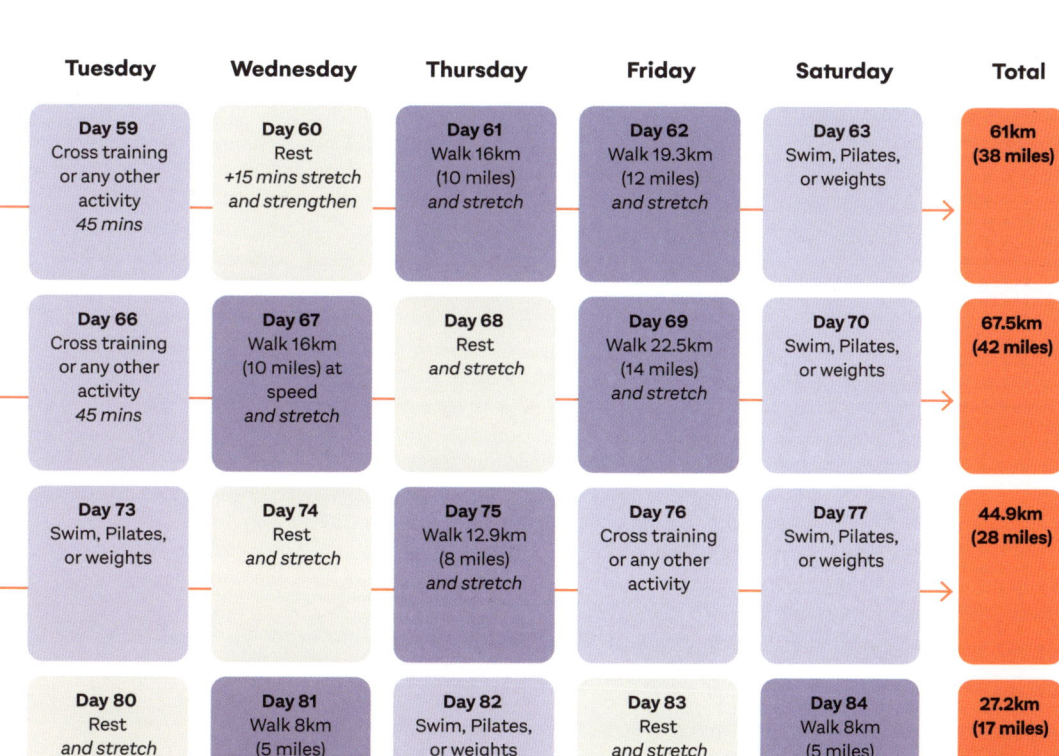

Other pages to help you: Interval training, see pp122–123 • Foods for health and fitness, see pp116–119 • Warming up and cooling down, see pp90–93 • Stretch and strengthen routine, see p95 • Cross training, see pp180-181 • Competitive race walking, see pp136–137 • Marathons, see pp162–167

Key — Walk days — Rest days — Other activity days

Tuesday	Wednesday	Thursday	Friday	Saturday	Total
Day 59 Cross training or any other activity 45 mins	Day 60 Rest +15 mins stretch and strengthen	Day 61 Walk 16km (10 miles) and stretch	Day 62 Walk 19.3km (12 miles) and stretch	Day 63 Swim, Pilates, or weights	61km (38 miles)
Day 66 Cross training or any other activity 45 mins	Day 67 Walk 16km (10 miles) at speed and stretch	Day 68 Rest and stretch	Day 69 Walk 22.5km (14 miles) and stretch	Day 70 Swim, Pilates, or weights	67.5km (42 miles)
Day 73 Swim, Pilates, or weights	Day 74 Rest and stretch	Day 75 Walk 12.9km (8 miles) and stretch	Day 76 Cross training or any other activity	Day 77 Swim, Pilates, or weights	44.9km (28 miles)
Day 80 Rest and stretch	Day 81 Walk 8km (5 miles) and stretch	Day 82 Swim, Pilates, or weights	Day 83 Rest and stretch	Day 84 Walk 8km (5 miles) and stretch	27.2km (17 miles)

Cross training

The saying goes, "A change is as good as a rest", and this is certainly true for the body. Walking primarily works your calves, hamstrings, and glutes, so to give these muscles recovery time try activities that work other muscles, or that challenge the same muscles in a different way.

Any type of exercise is suitable for cross training, as long as it raises your heart rate. Don't feel restricted to the following list – the most important thing is enjoying the activity and being able to complete a minimum of 30 minutes in each session.

Swimming
Swimming is a good all-round activity that can relieve stress. It's cardiovascular, builds endurance, improves your posture, and tones muscle due to the water resistance. Try building up to 30 minutes of continuous swimming in a session, or try water aerobics, pool-walking, or pool-running. The latter two activities involve walking or running lengths of the pool. Or give interval training in the pool a go – it can be high energy so it's an excellent way to burn calories.

Cycling
Riding a bike will give a good aerobic workout, increase your levels of strength and stamina, and support your muscle function. As a non-impact sport, it specifically works the abductors, developing good balance and coordination. Be aware that cycling shortens calf muscles and walking lengthens them, so always fully stretch when moving from one discipline to the other.

There are many different types of bikes suitable for speed and touring, mountain bikes for off-road trails and orienteering, as well as racing bikes and tandems. Research different clubs and organizations to discover what type of cycling appeals to you.

Dancing
Depending on your choice of dance and how vigorous you are, dancing can develop overall body fitness, coordination, and balance. It is cardiovascular and puts your core stability to the test, working your abdominal obliques. It can be weight bearing and burn about 300 calories per hour, which is the same as walking or cycling. Whether it's salsa, jazz, belly, swing, hip-hop, tango, modern, or quick step, dancing is social and fun. To get the maximum benefit, dance for an hour, not forgetting a few stretches before and after.

Rollerblading
For an activity that can look so effortless, rollerblading burns up a surprisingly large amount of energy, especially when you are learning. It is tremendous for developing core stability and coordination, and it particularly works the muscles of the legs and glutes. Because a lot of your control and power comes from the lower body and knees, work at strengthening these muscles with lunges.

Pilates
Pilates is one of my favourites and perhaps the perfect companion to walking as it works on elongating, stretching, and strengthening your muscles. Created by Joseph Pilates, it follows

six key principles: centring, concentration, control, precision, breath, and flow. The sequences promote flexibility, balance, and strength, improving overall body function and awareness. It can be done on a mat, or on a reformer – a piece of equipment that adds resistance to the workout. There are now many different versions, so try a few classes and find one that works for you.

Kettlebells

Kettlebells come in a variety of weights and look like a cannonball with a handle. The beauty of this tool is that the weights can be tailored to suit all ages and fitness abilities, and offer endless variations of both cardio and strengthening workouts. It comes with a long list of all-round benefits. These include improving muscle tone, core strength, flexibility, balance, and not least of all, developing good posture. Once you have mastered the technique and know what you are doing, this is an easy workout to do at home. Ideally performed 2–3 times a week, even 5 minutes a day can reap benefits. To get started, find a reputable instructor to learn the technique.

In the gym

If you are looking for variety with your cross training options, access to experienced instructors, and sociability with like-minded people, then head to a gym. You will find everything you need for a workout, including cardio equipment such as treadmills, rowing machines, and spin bikes. A long list of classes should be at your disposal, from circuit training to kick boxing, Pilates to dance. You may even find some gyms have swimming pools and saunas.

Given that most treadmills are situated in front of mirrors, the gym is an ideal environment to work on correcting your posture and overall walking technique. With an instructor, you gain the advantage of expert guidance in creating a personalized fitness plan.

Overtraining

Sometimes trying to fit in an extreme walking programme, when you have other stresses in your life, can itself become stressful and lead to burnout. Overtraining syndrome occurs when the stress of repetitive or intense training and exercise such as back-to-back long walks affects your body's ability to recover.

The first stage of this syndrome is called overreaching. Rest, along with sleep and good nutrition is usually the answer. However, if it's ignored, it can lead to overtraining, from which recovery can take weeks or even months. Symptoms manifest themselves in different ways, but typically include fatigue, altered sleep patterns, unquenchable thirst, loss of appetite, muscle ache even after a light workout, depression or anxiety, feeling impatient or easily upset, and a high resting heart rate.

It's easier to prevent overtraining than to recover from it. However, you should always check that there are no other underlying health issues responsible for the symptoms you may be experiencing. Keep a log to monitor your progress. As with any intense training plan, include details of how you feel both physically and emotionally. Record your sleeping patterns and if necessary, how restful they are, and treat yourself to a massage or a week off from your training plan.

Walking log

Keeping a walking log can help you to track your progress and stay committed to your goal. Keep a record of when, where, how far, and at what pace you walk. Add in your thoughts on the walk, or any other detail that is important to you. Over time this will build a pattern of your fitness journey: identifying your strengths and weaknesses, what makes you feel good, and what doesn't. It can be a great motivational tool, helping you to look back when you feel discouraged, as well as to acknowledge your stepping stones towards successes.

Month no:

Date	Distance	Time	Calories/heart rate	Route	Comments

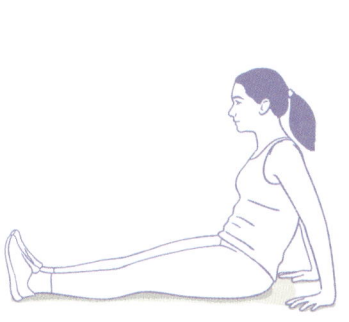
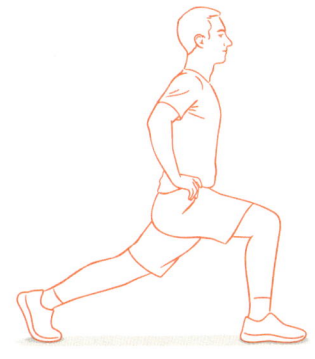

Month no:

Date	Distance	Time	Calories/heart rate	Route	Comments

Resources

Walk the Walk
Tel: 01483 741430
Email: info@walkthewalk.org
walkthewalk.org
For information on health, wellbeing and all types of walks and walking challenges.

Race Walking Association
www.racewalkingassociation.org.uk
For information and resources about the sport and the association.

The Ramblers' Association
Tel: 020 3961 3232
Email: ramblers@ramblers.zendesk.com
ramblers.org.uk
For details of local groups, events, and campaigns.

Go4awalk.com
Email: helpdesk@go4awalk.com
This website is excellent for walking and hiking information, and for providing maps of all areas within the UK.

Society for Barefoot Living
barefooters.org
Find out more from people who simply prefer to go barefoot.

British Orienteering Federation
The national body for orienteering in the UK.
britishorienteering.org.uk
Email: info@britishorienteering.org.uk
For a good explanation of orienteering, advice on clubs and associations, and national competitions.

Walkingworld
walkingworld.com
Access to hundreds of walks across the UK and Europe.

Nordicwalking.co.uk
For information on walks, instructors and local clubs.

Pilates.co.uk
Email: info@pilates.co.uk
For information on classes near you.

Strongfirst.com
Everything you need to know about getting stronger, including access to the best kettlebell instruction and classes.

Living Streets
livingstreets.co.uk
Email: info@livingstreets.co.uk
Working to support a safe environment on our streets to encourage people of all ages to get walking.

Goruck.eu
For information on rucking kit and communities worldwide.

RECOMMENDED READING

Erling Kagge, *Walking: One Step at a Time* (London: Penguin, 2020)

Caroline Idiens, *Fit at 50: Your Guide to a Stronger, Fitter, and Happier (Mid) Life in Just 6 Weeks* (London: DK Red, 2025)

James Nestor, *Breath* (London: Penguin, 2020)

Shane O'Mara, *In Praise of Walking* (London: Vintage, Penguin, 2019)

Annabel Streets, *52 Ways to Walk*, (London: Bloomsbury, 2023)

Ann Swanson, *Science of Yoga* (London: Dorling Kindersley, 2019)

References

Walking for fitness
Elena Barrera, "Walking workouts: 9 myths and facts to know", Everyday Health, 29 January, 2024, available at: https://www.everydayhealth.com/fitness/walking-workouts-myths-and-facts-to-know/

Malia Frey, "How to use interval walking for weight loss", Verywell fit, 3 August 2022, available at: https://www.verywellfit.com/how-to-use-interval-walking-to-lose-weight-3495456

Daniel Bubnis, "Need a change of pace? Try walking on an incline!", Healthline, 3 March 2021, available at: https://www.healthline.com/nutrition/walking-on-incline

Chris Napier, *Science of Running*, (London: Dorling Kindersley, 2020).

Walking for longevity
Katherine Schaeffer, "US Centenarian Population is projected to quadruple over the next 30 years", Pew Research Center, 9 January 2024, available at: https://www.pewresearch.org/short-reads/2024/01/09/us-centenarian-population-is-projected-to-quadruple-over-the-next-30-years/

Emily Abbate, "The Longest Living People in the World All Abide by the "Power 9" Rule", *GQ Magazine*, 26 February 2024, available at: https://www.gq.com/story/blue-zones-power-9

"Queen's research shows sedentary lifestyle linked to 70,000 deaths per year in the UK", Queen's University Belfast, available at: https://www.qub.ac.uk/News/Allnews/2019/sedentarylifestylelinkedto70000deathsperyearintheUK.html

David Pilbury, "Top tips for walking with arthritis", *Versus Arthritis*, 4 March 2024, available at:https://versusarthritis.org/news/2024/march/top-tips-for-walking-with-arthritis/

Laura Nathan-Garner, "Boost your walking workout to lower your cancer risk", MD Anderson Cancer Center, January 2025, available at: https://www.mdanderson.org/publications/focused-on-health/FOH-walking-workout.h10-1589835.html#:~:text=Walking%2C%20after%20all%2C%20can%20be,for%20breast%20and%20endometrial%20cancers

Karen Hallisey, "Doctor's Orders: Walk and Bike to Boost Your Immune System", UCLA Transportation, 23 February, 2021, available at: https://transportation.ucla.edu/blog/doctors-orders-walk-and-bike-your-way-better-immune-system

"12 Sedentary Lifestyle Statistics in 2021 That Will Get You off Your Chair", Ergonomic Trends, available at: https://ergonomictrends.com/sedentary-lifestyle-sitting-statistics/

Julie Corliss, "Revitalize your walking routine", Harvard Health Publishing, 1 February 2023, available at: https://www.health.harvard.edu/heart-health/revitalize-your-walking-routine#:~:text=Taking%20a%20daily%20walk%20is,30%25%2C%22%20says%20Dr

Walking for mental health
Alyssa Hunt, "The power of walking: steps to better health", Loma Linda University Health, 20 June 2024, available at: https://news.llu.edu/health-wellness/power-of-walking-steps-better-health#:~:text=Consistent%20walking%20can%20lower%20the,natural%20mood%20lifters%2C%20Studer%20says

"Mental Health Awareness Color And Its Impact", Social Recovery Center, 25 September 2024, available at: https://www.socialrecoverycenter.com/blog/mental-health-awareness-color#:~:text=Influence%20of%20Color%20on%20Mental%20Health,-Color%20has%20a&text=The%20presence%20of%20green%20can,and%20a%20sense%20of%20renewal

Lawrence Robinson, Jeanne Segal, and Melinda Smith, "The Mental Health Benefits of Exercise", Healthguide.org, available at: https://www.helpguide.org/wellness/fitness/the-mental-health-benefits-of-exercise

"Our top tips on connecting with nature to improve your mental health", Mental Health Foundation, 2021, available at: https://www.mentalhealth.org.uk/our-work/research/our-top-tips-connecting-nature-improve-your-mental-health

Tyler Wheeler, "Mental Benefits of Walking, WebMD, 28 February 2024, available at: https://www.webmd.com/fitness-exercise/mental-benefits-of-walking

"Barefoot grounding for managing my social anxiety", Anxiety NZ, available at: https://anxiety.org.nz/resources/barefoot-grounding-for-managing-my-social-anxiety#:~:text=It%20is%20based%20on%20the,energy%20is%20naturally%20re%2Dcharged

Walking at any age
"Walking - the benefits for older people", Better Health Channel, available at: https://www.betterhealth.vic.gov.au/health/healthyliving/Walking-the-benefits-for-older-people#bhc-content

Sara G Miller, "Pick Up the Pace: Walking Speed Linked with Heart Health in Older Adults", LiveScience, 19 November 2025, available at: https://www.livescience.com/52859-faster-longer-walking-heart-health.html

"A lack of physical activity is linked to high blood pressure, and being more active will lower your blood pressure", Blood Pressure UK, available at: https://www.bloodpressureuk.org/your-blood-pressure/how-to-lower-your-blood-pressure/healthy-living/exercise-physical-activity/

Jean-Charles Lebeau, "Cognitive Benefits of Physical Activity for Older Adults", American College of Sports Medicine (ACSM), 20 May 2022, available at: https://www.acsm.org/blog-detail/acsm-blog/2022/05/20/cognitive-benefits-physical-activity-older-adults

Walking for pregnancy
Jennifer Kelly Geddes, "Walking During Pregnancy", What to expect, 19 November 2021, available at: https://www.whattoexpect.com/pregnancy/keeping-fit/week-38/walk-it-off.aspx#benefits

Tracy Ward, *Science of Pilates*, (London: Dorling Kindersley, 2022).

Walking for children
"The Physiological Benefits Of Walking With Children", Kinder Pod, 10 February 2022, available at: https://kinderpod.com/blogs/news/the-physiological-benefits-of-walking-with-children?srsltid=AfmBOoq2BSjl1sjqIUyLDZtaKEPbCiSSTG_hi5b-WXecOBzTYVe55__X

Walking to heal
Carlolina Simioni, Giorgio Zauli, Alberto M Martelli, Marco Vitale, Gianni Sacchetti, Arianna Gonelli, Luca M Neri, "Oxidative stress: role of physical exercise and antioxidant nutraceuticals in adulthood and aging", National Library of Medicine, 30 March 2018, available at: https://pmc.ncbi.nlm.nih.gov/articles/PMC5908316/

Ronda Wendler, "Exercise during cancer treatment: 4 things to know", MD Anderson Cancer Center, 12 October 2022, available at: https://www.mdanderson.org/cancerwise/exercise-during-cancer-treatment--4-things-to-know.h00-159543690.html#:~:text=What%20they%20found%20left%20little,recover%20faster%20with%20fewer%20complications

"For Healing, Walk It Out", Harbin Clinic, 23 June 2023, available at: https://harbinclinic.com/blog/walkitout/#:~:text=Although%20after%20a%20hard%20workout,walking%20into%20your%20healing%20journey%3F

Stephen McMullan, Christine Nguyen, Dustin K Smith, "Can Walking Lower Blood Pressure in Patients With Hypertension?", American Family Physician, 2022, available at: https://www.aafp.org/pubs/afp/issues/2022/0100/p22.html#:~:text=The%20findings%20of%20this%20review,adult%20men%20and%20women%20with

Healthy choices
"Why 5 a day?", NHS, 12 July 2022, https://www.nhs.uk/live-well/eat-well/5-a-day/why-5-a-day/

Treadmill walking
Priyankaa Joshi, "I used an under-desk treadmill every day for 2 weeks – here's everything I learned", Women's Health, 13 August 2024, available at: https://www.womenshealthmag.com/uk/fitness/workouts/a41964659/under-desk-treadmill/

Jane McGuire, "The best under-desk treadmills 2024: tested and reviewed – walking while you work", Tom's Guide, 2 October 2024, available at: https://www.tomsguide.com/best-picks/best-under-desk-treadmills#section-best-folding-under-desk-treadmill

Barefoot walking
"Feel the earth beneath your feet – the benefits of Barefoot Walking", Combe Grove, available at: https://combegrove.com/health-and-wellbeing/2021/the-benefits-of-barefoot-walking/

Sara Lindberg, "Does Walking Barefoot Have Health Benefits?", Healthline, 8 March 2019, available at: https://www.healthline.com/health/walking-barefoot

Sandi Schwartz, "Discover the Mental Health Benefits of Walking Barefoot and Earthing", Ecohappiness Project, 26 May 2022, available at: https://ecohappinessproject.com/benefits-of-walking-barefoot/

Nordic walking
"The benefits of Nordic Walking", Nordic Walking UK, available at: https://nordicwalking.co.uk/benefits-of-nordic-walking/

"Nordic walking and poles", Fitwalk Ireland, available at: https://www.fitwalkireland.com/nordic-walking-poles

Korin Miller, "Nordic Walking Can Help Improve Heart Health – Here's How To Do It", Health, 16 September 2022, available at: https://www.health.com/news/nordic-walking-heart-health-benefits

Healthy walking
"Daily 11 minute brisk walk enough to reduce risk of early death", Research, University of Cambridge, 1 March 2023, available at: https://www.cam.ac.uk/research/news/daily-11-minute-brisk-walk-enough-to-reduce-risk-of-early-death

"5 surprising benefits of walking", Harvard Health Publishing, 7 December 2023, available at: https://www.health.harvard.edu/staying-healthy/5-surprising-benefits-of-walking

Index

A
abdominal breathing 101
abdominal muscles 29, 77
Achilles tendon massage 107
Achilles tendon stretch 87
active recovery 33
affirmations 103
age and walking 26
agility 8
alarms 54, 55
alcohol 21
ankles, massage 107
ankle stretch 70, 87
antioxidants 22
apps 17, 52
arms 64
arthritis 22, 32
asthma 50
athlete's foot 44

B
babies, walking with 29
back
 lower flexibility 8
 posture 60
backpacks 53, 128, 130
back stretch 89
back stretch roll down 92
balance 8
barefoot walking 24, 132–33
belly breathing 101
bird dog plank 82
black toenails 45
blisters 44
blood pressure see
 hypertension
Blue Zones 21
body awareness 104–05
body-scanning 104–05
Borg scale 10–11

bottled water 111
bras 48–49
breathing 98–101
buddies 13
Buettner, Dan 21
bum bags 47, 53, 54

C
caffeine 113, 117
calf muscles 70
calf stretch 87, 93
cancer 22, 23
cancer treatment 32
carbohydrates 116
carbonated water 111
cardiovascular health 22, 23, 26
centenarians 20
challenge walking 12, 31, 138–39, 168–73
change 105
charity challenges 12, 31, 138–39, 168–73
children 30–31
chiropodists 36
chronic diseases 32
climate and walking 50–51
clothing 46–49, 51, 128
coffee 113, 117
cognitive function 26
community 21
consistency 105
cooling down 90, 94, 105
core muscles 60, 61
core strength 8, 77, 80–83
corpse pose 93
cross training 105, 180–81
cycling 180

D
daily walking 12–13
daily walks, training plan 144–47
dancing 180
dehydration 17, 110
depression 25, 26
diabetes 23, 32
diaphragmatic breathing 101
diastasis rectus abdominis 29
diet, plant-based 21, 112, 116
distance
 children 30
 increasing 17
double leg stretch 78

E
earthing 24
electrolytes 110
endorphins 24, 25, 30, 140

F
fats, dietary 112
feet
 anatomy 132
 care 105 – 09
 massage 106–07
 size 37
filtered water 110
fingers, swollen 45
fitness
 heart rate 9
 testing 8, 56
 training plan 152–55
 ultra fitness 174–79
 walking 18
flexibility 8, 76
food
 antioxidants 22
 carbohydrates 116

energy boosting 118–19
fats 112
healthy choices 112–13
long-distance walking 117
plant-based diet 21, 112, 116
vitamins and minerals 114–15
walking supplies 31, 117
weight control 16, 17
footprint analysis 36
footwear 36–43, 105, 127–28, 133
Frieden, Thomas 32
fruit 113, 114
fundraising 138–39

G
gait 36–37, 132
geocaching 31
gloves 45, 47, 51
glucose 116
glycogen 116
goal setting 11
GPS 52
grounding 24
group walking 13, 25, 27
gym workouts 181

H
hamstring and calf stretch 87
"happy hormones" 24, 25
hats 47, 50, 51
healing 32
health and walking 140–41
health span 20
heart rate 9
heart-rate monitors 53
heat stroke/heat exhaustion 50
heels, slim 37
heel-to toe rock 72
hiking 126–27, 168–73
hiking boots 39
hip flexor stretches 86
Hippocrates 32

Holtz, Lou 11
humidity 50
hypertension 23, 26, 32, 33

I
ill-health prevention 140
immune system 22
ingrown toenails 45
injuries 44–45, 70, 72–73
insoles 36, 38
interval walking 17, 18, 122–23

J
juicing 115

K
kettebells 181
knee plank 81
knee to elbow plank 81
knee to nose plank 82

L
lacing techniques 42–43
layering clothes 46, 51
legs 62–63
lifestyles
  Power 9 21, 23
  sedentary 22–23
lifestyles, sedentary 77
long-distance walking 117, 168–73
longevity 20–23

M
mall walking 57
mantras 129
marathons 136–37, 162–67
massage, feet 106–07
meditation 128–29
meetings, walking 140
mental health 24–25
metabolism 17
mind 90
mind-body link 99
mindful walking 128–29

mindset 102–03
minerals 114–15
mineral water 111
minimalist shoes 133
mistakes in walking 68–69
monitoring, wearable tech 9, 17, 52–53
MoonWalk 139
motivation 11
muscles 19, 77

N
nature 24
neck stretch 84
negativity 102
neurotransmitters 23
night walking 55
Nordic walking 11, 134–35
nutrition see food

O
omega fatty acids 112
organic foods 113
orthotics 36, 38
osteoporosis 32
overtraining 181
oxygenated water 111

P
pace 16–17
pedometers 52
pelvic floor 29
Pilates 78–79, 180–81
plank exercises 80–83
planning routes 13, 55, 56–57
planning time for walking 12–13, 17, 140
plantar fasciitis 45
podiatrists 36
positivity 102–03
post-surgery walking 32
posture 60–69, 98, 104
Power 9 21, 23
power walking 10, 16, 18, 104
pregnancy 28–29

pronation 36, 70
protein 116
purified water 111
pursed lip breathing 100

Q
quad stretch 70

R
race walking 136–37
racewalking 11
recovery from illness 33
reflective clothing 47, 54, 55
resources 184
reverse plank 83
rhythmic breathing 100
road walking 122–23
rollerblading 180
route planning 13, 55, 56–57
rucking 18, 130–31

S
safety 54–55
sedentary lifestyles 22–23, 77
self-belief 103
shin splints 70, 72–73
shoes 36–43, 105, 127–28, 133
shoulder stretch 85
side rolls 88
side stitch 100
single straight leg stretch 79
sleep 25, 141, 181
smartphones 52, 54
smart watches 9, 17, 52–53
social circles 21
socks 38, 44, 49, 105
speed walking 137
sponsorship 138–39
sports bras 48–49
sprains 70, 72–73
spring water 111
stamina 156–61
standing hip flexor lunge 86
step counting 8, 17, 26, 53, 140

stitch 100
strains 70, 72–73
strength
  core strength 8, 77, 80–83
  daily routine 95, 105
  testing 8
  training plans 156–61
stress 21
stress reduction 25, 140
stretching
  beginners 78–79
  daily routine 95, 105
  flexibility 76
  full body 88–89
  lower body 86–87
  upper body 84–85
stride setting
  cold weather 50
  technique and flexibility 10–11
strolling 16
supination 36
supplements 114
swimming 180

T
teenagers 30
time to walk, finding 12–13, 17, 140
toddlers 23
toenails 45, 109
toes 37, 38
toe socks 49
trail walking 53
training plans
  daily walks 144–47
  long-distance walking 168–73
  marathons 162–67
  muscle strength and stamina 156–61
  ultra fitness 174–79
  walk yourself well 148–51
  weight control and fitness 152–55

treadmill walking 124–25, 181
tree (yoga) 91
tricep stretch 84

U
ultra fitness 174–79
under-desk treadmills 125
upper back stretch 85
urban walking 57

V
vegetables 113, 114
visualizations 103
vitamins 114–15

W
walking, fitness testing 8, 56
walking groups 13, 25, 27
walking log 182–83
walking poles 127, 134–35
Walk the Walk 139
wall sit 74
warming up 90, 94, 105
water 17, 51, 110–11
water holders 47, 53
wearable tech 9, 17, 52–53
weather forecasts 50
weight control 16–17, 152–55
weights 65, 130–31, 181
wind chill factor 51
Wright, Frank Lloyd 24

Y
yoga 87, 91, 93

Acknowledgements

This book has been created with love, care, and tremendous patience from all at DK for which I cannot ever thank them enough. In particular, I would like to thank Jasmin, Susan, and the wonderful design team, Barbara and Louise.

Thank you also to the many, many people I have met and walked with over the years. You have taught me all I know about walking, proving time and time again that a good walk can be the magical answer to almost everything. I would also like to thank my husband Guy, my daughter Raphaelle, and my family and my friends for their loving support, encouragement and even more patience.

Writing a book can be incredibly anti-social and demanding on all those around you. Last but not least I want to thank my mum, who unexpectedly slipped away while I was in the middle of writing. You always taught me that I could do anything I put my mind to … thanks Mum, this one's for you!

PUBLISHER'S ACKNOWLEDEGMENTS
The publisher would like to thank Kathy Steer for proofreading; Ruth Ellis for indexing; Aditya Katyal for data clearance; and everyone involved in creating the first edition of this book.

DISCLAIMER
Neither the publisher nor the author is engaged in rendering professional advice or services to the individual reader. The ideas, procedures, and suggestions contained in this book are not intended as a substitute for consulting with your doctor or a professional. All matters regarding your health require supervision. Neither the author nor the publisher shall be liable or responsible for any loss or damage allegedly arising from any information or suggestion in this book.

CREDITS
20 United Nations (UN): From Department of Economic and Social Affairs,; "World Population Prospects: 2015 Revision ©2015 United Nations. Used with the permission of the United Nations (br). **22 Copyright Clearance Center - Rightslink:** Oxford University Press-American Journal of Epidemiology / Data used from-Alpa V. Patel, Leslie Bernstein, Anusila Deka, Heather Spencer Feigelson, Peter T. Campbell, Susan M. Gapstur, Graham A. Colditz, Michael J. Thun, Leisure Time Spent Sitting in Relation to Total Mortality in a Prospective Cohort of US Adults, American Journal of Epidemiology, Volume 172, Issue 4, 15 August 2010, Pages 419–429, https://doi.org/10.1093/aje/kwq155 (br). **24 PNAS:** Data Used From-Bratman, G. N., Hamilton, J. P., Hahn, K. S., Daily, G. C., & Gross, J. J. (2015). Nature experience reduces rumination and subgenual prefrontal cortex activation. Proceedings of the National Academy of Sciences, 112(28), 8567-8572. https://doi.org/10.1073/pnas.1510459112 (br). **33 Copyright Clearance Center - Rightslink:** John Wiley and Sons / Data Used From-Lee LL, Mulvaney CA, Wong YK, Chan ESY, Watson MC, Lin HH. Walking for hypertension. Cochrane Database of Systematic Reviews 2021, Issue 2. Art. No.: CD008823. DOI: 10.1002/14651858.CD008823.pub2. (b)

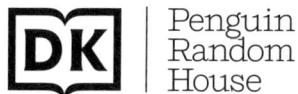

Senior Acquisitions Editor Zara Anvari
Editor Jasmin Lennie
Senior Designer Barbara Zuniga
Senior Production Editor David Almond
Senior Production Controller Kariss Ainsworth
Publishing Co-ordinator Emily Cannings
DTP & Design Co-ordinator Heather Blagden
Art Director Maxine Pedliham
Publishing Director Stephanie Jackson

Editorial Susan McKeever
Design Louise Evans
Illustration Andrew Torrens

First published in Great Britain in 2025 by
Dorling Kindersley Limited
20 Vauxhall Bridge Road,
London SW1V 2SA

The authorised representative in the EEA is
Dorling Kindersley Verlag GmbH. Arnulfstr. 124,
80636 Munich, Germany

Copyright © 2025 Dorling Kindersley Limited
A Penguin Random House Company
Text copyright © Nina Barough 2025;
Nina Barough has asserted her right to be
identified as the author of this work.

10 9 8 7 6 5 4 3 2 1
001-345510-May/2025

All rights reserved.
No part of this publication may be reproduced, stored in or introduced into a retrieval system, or transmitted, in any form, or by any means (electronic, mechanical, photocopying, recording, or otherwise), without the prior written permission of the copyright owner.

A CIP catalogue record for this book
is available from the British Library.
ISBN: 978-0-2417-2605-1

Printed and bound in China
www.dk.com

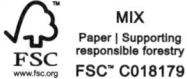

This book was made with Forest Stewardship Council™ certified paper – one small step in DK's commitment to a sustainable future. Learn more at **www.dk.com/uk/information/sustainability**

About the author

Nina Barough is the founder and CEO of cancer charity Walk the Walk. She has always been intrigued by the relationship and balance between what we eat, how active we are, and the impact that has both physically and mentally on our wellbeing. She finds walking a wonderful way of helping to achieve this balance, as well as maintaining her passion for good health and fitness. She has been a vegetarian from a young age, and has studied massage and Reiki healing.

Nina started walking in earnest following a dream that she power walked the New York City Marathon in a bra to raise money for breast cancer. Although she knew nothing about breast cancer, or marathons, she loved the idea of a weekend in New York and went on to power walk the marathon. Only eight weeks later, she discovered she had breast cancer herself. This ultimately led to Walk the Walk being formed and becoming a much-loved and well-supported charity that has encouraged more than half a million people to start walking their way to better health. Nina has walked over 150 marathons, numerous half marathons, and has led multiple treks in different parts of the world from the sub-Arctic to Peru.

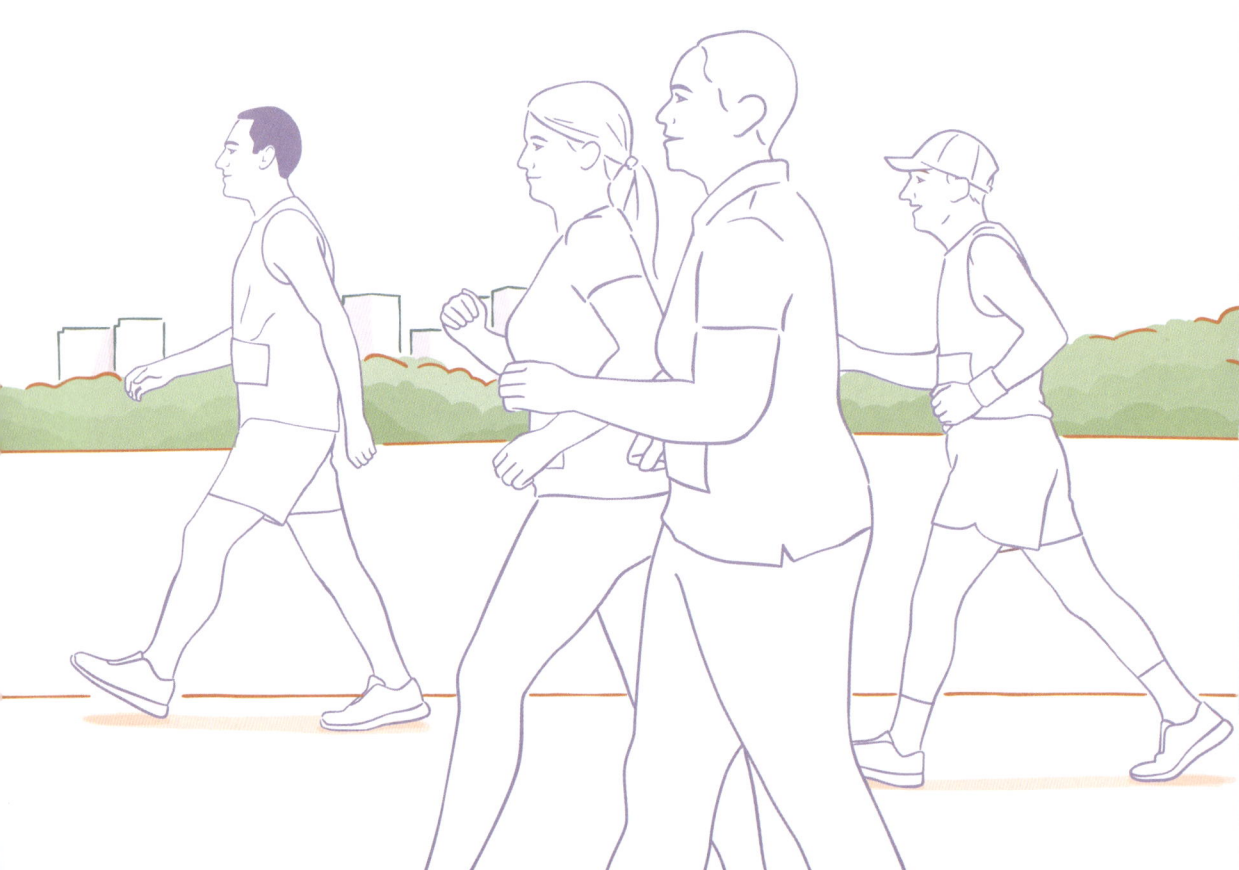